RUN DOWN

RUN DOWN

An Endurance Athlete's Race Against Chronic Fatigue

MICHAEL GALLAGHER, MD

Foreword by
Olympian Kara Goucher

Run Down

Cover design: Lauria Fiverr.com/lauria
Cover photo: Courtesy of REVEL Race Series

Paperback ISBN 979-8-9857790-0-4
Hardback ISBN 979-8-9857790-1-1
ASIN B09ML79RDW (ebook)

Printed in the United States of America

mdgallagher.com

609737

To Melissa: For loving and caring and cooking for the kids and me more than we could ever ask. For checking in on how I was feeling thousands of times. For taking up the slack and guiding the family through the toughest times.

To Owen and Reese: You have witnessed your father go through hell with a front-row seat, and you never complained that I wasn't the dad I used to be. Please don't read this until you're old enough to understand.

I love you, family.

For the millions missing.

It occurred to me that there was no difference between men, in intelligence or race, so profound as the difference between the sick and the well.

F. Scott Fitzgerald
The Great Gatsby

Contents

Author's Note

This book contains recollections of events and experiences from my personal life. Although all these stories are true, I have accurately recreated the events to the best of my ability based on my memories. I recognize that some may remember these experiences differently by the individuals mentioned herein, and I do not intend harm or maliciousness toward anyone in these recollections. In some cases, names and identifying details have been changed to protect the identities of the individuals.

I have used the technique of reconstructed dialogue to recreate the feelings and meanings of real events. The dialogue herein is accurate to the best of my recollection, though not verbatim.

Ultimately, this book is about my life. It is not meant to elucidate a pathway to diagnose, deal with, or treat myalgic encephalomyelitis (ME), addiction, COVID, or any other malady. Because it is a memoir, there is a lot about me. Although a portion of the book deals with my life before my illness and diagnosis, the events described therein contributed to where and who I am today. Regardless, I have shared my experience to provide insight into what it is like to live with ME and to help the world better understand what ME is and what it does to people and families.

Foreword by Olympian Kara Goucher

As a professional runner and Olympian, I have always been able to rely on my body. I've made a living out of racing endurance events and pushing myself to the extreme limits. There is a great empowerment in the suffering, in feeling the pain, yet being able to continue toward the finish line. It is addictive, and it has a way of becoming a part of your personality. It can define who you are and what your daily life looks like.

But what if that was taken away in an instant? What if there was no finish line to get to? Instead of running a marathon, you struggle to get out of bed, to perform the simplest tasks in life. Everyone knows you as superhuman, yet you find yourself at war with your own body, unable to do the things that used to be routine, the things we take for granted.

Imagine the frustration and fear. You are living someone else's life.

For our friend Michael Gallagher, that became a reality.

Michael takes us through his astonishing journey in *Run Down*, a touching memoir of a life filled with triumph and tragedy. An endurance athlete who races marathons and Ironman triathlons, Michael thrives on challenges. As an orthopedic surgeon, he not only tests the limits of his body in the physical space; he also pushes himself mentally. He is a father, an athlete, and a doctor. He is as active as anyone I know. But when he starts to grapple with a mysterious illness, it leads him down a long and at times harrowing path. As he navigates his symptoms and the loss of the ability to do the things he loves, he struggles to find a diagnosis. No one seems to be able to pinpoint what is going on with him, and he continues to suffer as the life he cherishes seems to slip away.

Worse yet, after he finally receives a diagnosis, Michael faces a new round of challenges. Once an incredible athlete, he now fears the stigma he faces telling the world he has chronic fatigue/myalgic encephalomyelitis (ME), an illness so maligned in his profession that he hides the truth, fearing unfair judgment from his patients and colleagues alike. He knows his partners will look at him differently. And yet he pushes on. He learns to live with ME, and he begins to share his difficult experiences and the lessons he has learned from them in an open and honest fashion, displaying what vulnerability really is.

Run Down is an incredible read whether you are an athlete, are someone struggling through tough times, or are just looking for meaning in life. The pain Michael has fought through is unfathomable. But for me, this story is about so much more. We all suffer in our own battles, wondering who believes us, who will be there for us. Most of the time we hold it all in, fearing judgment from our family, close friends, and peers. That is not what Michael did. He is living bravely, trying to break the stereotypes he faces in an effort to educate all of us and change the way we think about chronic illness. Yes, his struggle is with ME, but we all have our own private battles. These may be battles that we are embarrassed about, that we question ourselves over, and that leave us with shame. Michael has felt all of that, yet he pushes on to raise awareness and teach those around him. He is willing to open up to make the path easier and more welcoming for future men and women who face a similar fate.

In reading *Run Down*, we begin to examine ourselves. We scrutinize our own prejudices. We think about how we look at the world, and how we could change for the better. As Michael bravely opens up about the hardest time in his life, we see his struggle in ourselves. We see how to survive difficult times, how to rise up, and how to look out and care for others.

Michael Gallagher has left us with a memoir that will continue to sit with us after we finish the last page. Yes, we learn a lot about the diagnosis of ME and what it means, its unique challenges and difficulties. But we also are inspired to take action in our own lives, to listen to others, to learn from their experiences. At a time when the world can feel divided, we are reminded that we all have similar fears and similar rough patches in life. *Run Down* leaves us inspired to listen to our bodies, to take care of those around us and ourselves. From it, we can learn to heal in every sense of the word if we lend our hearts and minds to Michael's experiences put here in writing. The takeaways are endless and leave us with a new sense of our own strength.

-KG

Prologue—Boston

When the first bomb detonated on Boylston Street, I was getting into a cab two blocks away. As I shut the door, chaos reigned at the finish line of the Boston Marathon as one homemade pressure-cooker bomb exploded, followed thirteen seconds later by another, killing three innocent people and wounding two hundred sixty-four more. It was April 15, 2013, a day that would forever change thousands of lives and the way that America would perceive the Boston Marathon, and all mass spectator events to an extent.

Fourteen months later, another bomb of sorts would explode inside me and rip apart my life. That bomb went off in a place called the Badlands. I would never see another Boston Marathon start line again once it blasted through me.

That bomb was chronic fatigue syndrome. It is one of the most disregarded, misunderstood, debilitating illnesses in the world—so much so that the words *chronic fatigue syndrome* have a stigma attached to them. That stigma is at its worst inside the medical community. I should know. I am an orthopedic surgeon.

JUST AN HOUR BEFORE THE EXPLOSIONS, I RAN PAST THE site where the bombs went off and across the iconic blue-and-yellow finish line indelibly painted on Boylston Street. Years prior, my marathon time would've put me there right at the time of the attack. But over the past decade, I spent countless early mornings running more than ten thousand miles to qualify for Boston, finishing my first crack at it in three hours and ten minutes.

Shivering and feeling faint, I made my way through the eternally long finisher's corral and did a U-turn back toward the Westin Hotel, where I would meet my wife, my sister, and a few friends. Exhausted runners shuffled tentatively around the sidewalks as far as the eye could see, wrapped in foil blankets, wearing tiny nylon running shorts above bare, sinewy, goosebump-riddled legs.

Boston is the Woodstock of running, where people get high on adrenaline and bragging rights about finish times. I was no different from the others who had finished already, feeling a bit high myself. It was my first time running Boston—a lifelong goal—and a sense of triumph embraced me. What a memorable experience it would be. Only the whole world would remember this day. They would watch live streams of the following days, as well, as the intense and terrifying manhunt ensued for the two brothers who perpetrated the act of domestic terrorism. The entire city was on notice, and the term *Boston Strong* was born.

THE LEAD-UP TO MY FIRST BOSTON MARATHON HAD BEEN perfect, if not poetic. After nearly two decades of running for fun or to cure a hangover, I joined a running group a few years before I qualified for Boston. When I joined the group, my required qualifying time sat at three hours, fifteen minutes, but my best marathon time was nineteen minutes slower than that—a difference of more than forty seconds per mile. I figured at that time if I could just keep running that pace until I turned fifty—more than a dozen years away—I would make it. The alternative was to get significantly faster.

With the help of twice-weekly group workouts that pushed me to the point of wanting to vomit and a new group of friends who loved to run at 5:00 a.m. before work, I began to get faster. Eventually, I got fast enough to likely qualify for Boston. I could feel the excitement building within me.

Running Boston was a badge of honor that I felt would make me be able to say I was a real runner. Despite being a surgeon and having made it through grueling training programs at prestigious universities, it became a goal for me to identify myself as an athlete. I had finished two Ironman triathlons at that point, but I did so by never giving up, not by being particularly fast—a lesson I would draw upon in my darkest days. But there was something about being in my running group that finally pushed me to train for speed and try to reach Boston.

A few years earlier, my wife Melissa and I lived just a mile from the Boston Marathon course in the town of Newton with her parents during my fellowship at Harvard. I ran on sections of the course repeatedly, but I never saw the whole course nor was I able to watch the race in person—I was working on Patriots' Day that April when we lived in Massachusetts. But just living there and running in Newton got me thinking more than I ever had about the race. I had always wanted to experience running Boston, but it seemed out of reach.

As I tried to qualify by running a couple of marathons, I got my time down to three hours, twenty minutes. If I could repeat that performance a year later, it would mean I would qualify in the forty- to forty-four-year-old age group, which required a slower time than the thirty-five- to thirty-nine-year-old age group I had been in. I had it in the bag. I already knew I was capable of running the right time; I just needed to do so one measly year later. Boston had other ideas.

Because of the race's growing popularity, the Boston Athletic Association, the group that organizes the race, lowered the qualifying times for all age groups. My new forty- to forty-four-year-old age group now required a three-hour, fifteen-minute time. Dammit. I was back where I started. *Was that even possible for me to run?* I wondered. I had to. I felt it was my destiny.

I was scheduled to run the Poconos marathon in May 2012, just a few months before I would turn forty. A Boston qualifier, Pocono was known to be a fast course at relatively low altitude—an advantage for a runner like me coming from Boulder, where we would train between five thousand and eight thousand feet of elevation, routinely. I set my sights on going under three hours, fifteen minutes, and zero seconds, the slowest allowable time for me to be accepted to Boston.

In the year leading up to the Pocono marathon, I logged more than two thousand miles of running. The actual marathon training block itself took place in the dead of winter, which often meant running in the snow with frozen hands and toes, and a headlamp lighting the way through the dark hours of the morning. Many times, I would return home with frozen eyelashes and beard, the ice not fully melting until the hot water hit my face in the shower. The cold rivulets of snowmelt running down my neck and onto my chest were a satisfying feeling of early morning accomplishment.

In contrast to the cold winter training I had done, the day of the race in the Poconos was particularly warm, which is rarely welcomed by marathoners. Data show that the ideal temperature for racing is between 50 and 62 degrees. This day would reach more than 80.

I could feel the heat before the race even began. I was initially distracted by the excitement of the gun going off, being in the midst of a crowd of electrified runners, all of whom likely had high hopes for their performance that day, despite the weather. In the first mile I passed a woman running in a short plaid skirt that bounced rhythmically with each stride, revealing her bare bottom as the back of the skirt floated up and her feet landed back on the ground. I slowed momentarily, taking a closer look and thinking for a second that I was hallucinating. Despite the distraction, I kept moving, holding the pace I wanted but feeling like I was putting in more effort than the times on my watch were telling me. I kept trying to decide if taking the shortest route through the long winding turns in the road was a better option than staying on whichever part of the course offered the most shade from the hot sun. I hit the halfway mark forty seconds slower than I had hoped for, but I was still optimistic. I picked up the pace between miles thirteen and eighteen to give myself a little buffer for the end, constantly checking my splits on my Garmin.

At mile nineteen a woman ahead of me decided it was too hot for her and urged me to "give up on any time goals you have on a day like today" as I passed her. I entertained the idea briefly, but knew I had not trained for years to give up in the last eight miles. I was willing to test my mettle, at least for a little longer, for the sake of Boston.

At every aid station, I poured water down my throat and on my head. I was no longer able to pick up the pace, and at mile twenty-four I saw the bright pink shirt of the 3:15 pacer pass me. Earlier in the race I saw him and hoped that if I ever encountered him again, it would be at the twenty-six-mile mark, suggesting I was about to meet my goal.

The pacer ran by me all alone. Not one of the dozens of hopeful runners that accompanied him for the first half was still with him. As he moved ahead, I realized I was literally watching my Boston Marathon qualification run away from me. I tried desperately to speed up by fifteen seconds per mile and suddenly felt dizzy, my vision getting dark as if I'd entered a total solar eclipse. I could feel myself starting to wobble, then stumble, so I quickly slowed back down, regaining my balance and pushing on with a steadier, albeit stiff, gait. I hit mile twenty-six with ninety seconds left to get to the finish line in time. I was struggling to push on even with so little left to go. It felt like it was 100 degrees in the shade.

The finish line sat on the south end of the town's high school track, and as I set foot onto the grippy, rubber surface, I saw the pink shirt crossing the finish line, noticing that I still had forty-five seconds to make it more than halfway around the oval. Having done countless intervals on the track, I knew that I had to be sprinting like a horse coming down the homestretch in the hunt for the Triple Crown for me to make it to Boston.

Just weeks prior in the Kentucky Derby, I'll Have Another pulled out a win in the final furlong, clearly beating Bodemeister, but for this marathon, we'd have to go to the photo finish. I crossed the line with the race clock reading 3:15:10 and the announcer calling my name. My official time, called the chip time, the one that the Boston Marathon cares about, would depend on exactly how much time had elapsed from the time the gun went off until I crossed the official start line; races don't start the clock for runners until they cross the timing mat, which is measured by a chip on each runner's race number.

My watch said 3:15:02. I knew I had started my watch just a moment before I hit the timing mat at the start line. I now hoped that my chip time would read 3:15:00 and not 3:15:01, which would keep me out of Boston.

I actually felt great after finishing, proud that I'd hung in there for the end of such a hard race. For miles, my brain and body were telling me to slow down, but my heart would not let it happen. I was happy to have a new personal best marathon time and was thinking that at least it would be one hell of a story if I missed it by one second. I thought of every moment in the race in which I'd possibly squandered a second. My inhaler had fallen on the ground twice, and it took me ten seconds or so to pick it up each time. I fumbled a cup at a water stop. Another runner had cut me off, causing me to stop abruptly.

Then I thought of all the times I didn't stop. I wanted nothing more than to walk up the steep hill near mile twenty-two as the heat intensified. But I did not. I had to pee incredibly badly since mile six and made myself promise after promise that I would stop later. But I did not. I felt I should walk after I became dizzy and things got dark. But I did not. If I missed it by one second, so be it.

I walked back to the hotel, stopping for food and fluids at a gas station nearby. With a small twist of irony, the Garmin watch I had been obsessing over for 26.2 miles suddenly fell off my wrist and onto the glossy tile floor of the store as the pin in the band broke. I thought maybe it was a sign—of what I wasn't sure.

I called Melissa.

"I don't know if I made it," I told her. "It was really close."

"I know how much this means to you. I'm sure you made it."

"I don't know. Missing it by one second would be nuts, but there's nothing I can do about it now."

I showered, then drove back to the finish line, parking close enough that my blistered feet could tolerate the walk in flip-flops. As I got there, I looked for the times to be posted so I wouldn't have to wait until after my flight home to check online. As I scanned the wall, I found my name

MICHAEL GALLAGHER

SEVENTY-EIGHTH PLACE

CLOCK TIME 3:15:12

CHIP TIME 3:14:58

I made it. I fucking made it. I got choked up for a minute, nearly weeping as I happily shuffled back to my rental car.

As memorable as that day was, Boston would be even more so, but for more tragic reasons.

The start of the race is done in corrals of a thousand entrants clustered into three waves of nine thousand or so runners who set out in separate groups. The course, I quickly discovered, is particularly narrow early on, making it very difficult to move ahead in the large pack. Worse, Boston is known to have many bandits—people running the race without being registered—making it even more crowded. To boot, the first few miles are steeply downhill, enough to trash a runner's quads and make the hills later on in the race particularly difficult. But considering the fierce gale and torrential rain I'd run through in the California International Marathon just four months before, and my seventy-mile-a-week training throughout the bitter Colorado winter, I was not deterred.

As I moved through the throngs of runners, my eyes stayed focused on the feet and legs in front of me, looking for gaps that I could surge through to zig and zag my way past several thousand people by the finish. Before I knew it, I had run more than half the course and barely seen any of the towns we ran through. I stopped at mile sixteen to see my family cheering wildly for me, getting a big hug and kiss from my wife before heading up the first of the Newton hills. The last-minute decision for my wife and kids to spectate near her parents' home rather than at the finish line is one that may have altered the course of our lives forever, given the tragic events that unfolded there.

THE WORLD WOULD REMEMBER THE BOSTON bombing FOR years to come, but there would be no such tucket about the day the bomb went off inside me. It took another fourteen months for it to detonate. After I finished my first Boston Marathon, I went on to race Ironman Florida in November 2013, where I broke eleven hours, running a sub-four-hour marathon to complete the race—a significantly faster and smoother campaign than my first two Ironman finishes. I followed that up twenty-four weeks later with 2014's Boston Marathon on April 21—a day when we honored the victims of the year prior, running tall and proud to show the rest of the world that *Boston Strong* meant something real. It was one of the most amazing race experiences of my life, standing at the start in Hopkinton as we held a moment of silence, then staring skyward in awe as Blackhawk helicopters flew over, displaying America's military might.

I had hopes of running around three hours and three minutes that year, but as I warmed up the day before the race, my body felt heavy. Something was slightly off. Still, I powered through the toughest marathon of my life, besting my time from the year before by a mere ninety seconds. Despite that heavy feeling, I felt like I recovered in time for an upcoming mountain bike trip, not knowing what lay ahead.

What happened next in the Badlands would destroy the identity I had made for myself in Boston and make my life a living hell.

The events that unfolded there led me on a harrowing seven-year journey that culminated in me being bedridden, unable to work or care for myself, and wondering if I was going to survive. During the scariest part of my illness and the coinciding COVID-19 pandemic, I was finally diagnosed with chronic fatigue syndrome after far too long of not knowing what was happening to my body.

Chronic fatigue syndrome is now commonly referred to by patient groups and a growing part of the medical field as myalgic encephalomyelitis, or ME, though it has gone through multiple name changes over the years, including systemic exertional intolerance disease (SEID) and chronic fatigue and immune dysfunction syndrome (CFIDS).

No matter the name, confusion prevails. ME is an invisible illness. There are no lab tests to definitively diagnose it. Nor is there an agreed-upon treatment regimen or cure. Research has been scarce at best.

Getting diagnosed is incredibly difficult and commonly takes years, as it did for me. Many are never properly diagnosed, and diagnosis does not often provide a clear path to recovery. People with ME suffer intense bouts of illness after physical, mental, or emotional exertion. ME causes energy crashes that keep people from being able to live a normal life. Patients can have a spectrum of symptoms ranging from mild to severe. Some cases are catastrophic enough to cause people to be bedbound for months, years, or even decades. The stark reality is that for many patients with ME, working is impossible—and that is exactly what happened to me. It has also happened to a new wave of patients who have symptoms eerily similar to ME after COVID-19 infection. These are the COVID long haulers.

For a very active athlete and surgeon like me, developing ME has meant an end to my life as I knew it. For years after the Badlands, I was unwilling to accept the unimaginable changes that took place. Facing challenges in life beyond our control is a universal truth of the human condition. My illness, the death of a close friend, and the COVID-19 pandemic are three of the most striking examples of this in my life. Ironically, these events have also allowed me to realize that my identity and happiness are not staked in my marathon times or my job title and that like many before us have done, we are capable of accepting that which is beyond our control. I learned this lesson only after getting to the point of nearly giving up on life completely. The kid who wouldn't stop no matter the temperature or difficulty of the race found himself ready to call it quits.

Chapter 1

This Isn't Over

I grew up in what many would consider an all-American family. My parents, Denny and Pat, both grew up in New Jersey. They were relatively young when they had children, my mother having my sister Kelly at twenty-four and Kristi at twenty-seven. Last came my twin brother, Kevin, and me, three years later. We were towheaded, cute kids who were decently intelligent, especially the girls. My parents both had dark brown hair, so the four of us being blond was an unusual contrast.

My mother stayed home with us until Kevin and I attended junior high school, when she returned to work as a secretary at the high school right next door. She and my father met at a pharmaceutical company, where she was a secretary and he was a forklift operator in the warehouse.

My mother's career ambition was to be a secretary. She had all the smarts in the world, but unlike her brothers, who attended Ivy League schools, she was never made to believe she should do more. The private women's liberal arts school she started after high school lacked a good secretarial program, so after just one year, she moved back home and transferred to a secretarial school, commuting there with a pretty, outgoing woman named Mary, who would eventually wed her youngest brother, Larry.

When my mother and father met, Denny was a good-looking guy with a modicum of joie de vivre and a ripe sense of humor. My mother soon became pregnant, and her initial reaction was to go it on her own. So with her parents' help, she arranged to go to the home for unwed women far away in Indianapolis. My father, however, refused to let her go and demanded that they marry. Thus, with a tiny gathering of family and my mother dressed in a pantsuit, they wed on April 3, 1966. My parents always told us that they were married for one year longer than they were, lest we do the math that proved that their first daughter was conceived before the wedding. My father never admitted the truth to us kids by refusing to discuss it when we were old enough to ask about the apparent discrepancy.

Denny continued to work his way up the ladder, making his way into a warehouse management position. He found a better job at a rival pharmaceutical company and slowly advanced his career. Having married, divorced, and dropped out of college by nineteen, Denny lacked the credentials to continue his upward mobility, so he began attending night classes while working days. Nearly twelve years after his college career began in northern West Virginia, he graduated with a bachelor's degree in economics, with two children and two more on the way. From there his career flourished, and our family upgraded from a tiny three-bedroom house and a Volkswagen Beetle to a four-bedroom colonial and a Ford Country Squire station wagon equipped with fold-up seats in the back for the twins.

In many ways, my dad was a larger-than-life figure. He stood six feet three and was 265 pounds at his heaviest. He chomped cigars and drove a deep-blue 1971 Cadillac Eldorado convertible. He was a real-life Boss Hogg minus the steer horns on his hood. I was asked more than once if he played professional football. He could be charismatic and engaging at times, aloof and cynical at others.

Denny coached our baseball and hockey teams when we were kids. It was sometimes torturous. He could be short-tempered when he saw something he disliked. He had expectations that my brother and I would be something we obviously were not, though we weren't quite sure what that was.

"They don't seem to even care about baseball when they're out there," he would rant to my mother. "They run out of the dugout and jump off the pitcher's mound like a couple of idiots."

Afterward, my mother would come talk to us. "Your father wants you to try harder. It's embarrassing for him."

Denny became increasingly angry as my childhood progressed, aiming his paroxysmal ire at my brother and me far more than at our sisters. I don't remember him being angry much before I turned eight. That August, in 1980, we moved to Stony Brook, Long Island. He was offered a job as vice president at a plant there, a subsidiary of his current company.

We lived on Long Island for just seventeen months. During that time my father had fits of rage over things like a scratch on his car or his tools disappearing or being broken, although he never seemed to have much use for them. He resorted to knocking Kevin's and my heads together by grabbing our hair, kicking at us as we ran away or reaching from the front seat of the car to squeeze our thighs in what he called a horse bite. If we really pissed him off, he would pull the car over to teach us a lesson, dragging us out to express his displeasure.

He was fired from his job by a boss that he would later testify against on behalf of the company. His boss had terminated several employees, including my father, and replaced them with his cronies in an act of blatant nepotism. I remember my father coming home with a cardboard box full of his personal items and telling my mother that he had lost his job. My mother was incredulous. Her mother had died just months before, and now her husband was out of work. Being kids, we were insensitive to the matter. My brother and I took the gavel off a plaque he had been awarded and repeatedly slammed it on the table, mimicking the actions of a judge and saying, "You're fired!"

My father paradoxically laughed, which only encouraged us to do it more until it finally enraged him. For the next six months, Denny was at home every morning, sitting at the breakfast table before school. He grew a shitty beard, commented on our table manners, and gave Kevin and me a hard time about our penmanship.

"Your words are too close together!" he would shout. "I want you to put your finger down on the paper after each sentence. That's how much space you have to have between every word."

When is he going back to work? I wondered.

When we left for Long Island, I was slated to go into the gifted and talented program in third grade. When we got back to New Jersey in the middle of fourth grade, I was behind the average student. Somewhere along the way in Long Island I lost a step.

My third-grade teacher at Setauket Elementary was Mrs. Dawe. She wore a tight perm atop a face marked with angular features and dark eyes. Her Long Island accent was so thick that I thought her name was Mrs. Door for most of third grade. Mrs. Dawe would discipline kids by physical means—something I was only used to at home. I responded by zoning out. I missed homework assignments. Worse, I stole other children's work and put my name on it, pleading ignorance when I was caught. I loved the kids in my neighborhood, but I didn't love school. I was elated when we left.

Dissatisfied with the job prospects he found on Long Island, my father sold our house and moved us back to the town we had left in New Jersey just a year and a half before. Hopewell Township consists of three towns—Pennington, Titusville, and Hopewell—that in 1980 had a grand total of under ten thousand people spread out over fifty-nine square miles. Phone numbers were exchanged between people as four digits, assuming that the other person understood the first three numbers were 737. An area code was only used for a long-distance call, something Denny certainly was not willing to pay for.

Kevin and I were going back to the school where our two best friends in the world were when we left Long Island. Liam McCallister was one grade below us, and Luke Phillips was one below him. We lived three doors down from the Phillipses for the first four years of my life. They were like a second set of parents to Kevin and me throughout our childhood—and still are. Charlotte and Oliver McCallister were from England. Oliver was a scientist with a dry sense of humor and an even temper. Liam, Kevin, and I would spend hours imitating the McAllisters' British accents and saying things to them like, "You bloody fat cow," to get a laugh.

We settled in a bastardized Dutch Colonial house in Titusville, a tri-level of sorts with ample property and a five-hundred-acre field of corn and soybeans behind it. Across the street was a horse farm and a house whose owners maintained that George Washington had slept there, just as many others in our town claimed of their homes. Each Christmas Day, our town held a reenactment of Washington crossing the Delaware River in a rowboat from Pennsylvania into Titusville. The thirty-five-hundred-acre Washington Crossing State Park was just a mile from our house and extended down to the river, both sources of endless adventure for us as kids.

Between our house and the park was Bear Tavern Elementary School, where we had attended kindergarten through second grade and would resume our studies midway through fourth grade until junior high in seventh grade. Denny found a job again with his old company, but his new boss would prove to be his nemesis. He was overbearing, unpleasant, and had a bone to pick with my father. As Denny's relationship with his boss spoiled, his weight ballooned and his mood darkened. I heard his boss's name uttered nearly every night at the dinner table. My mother would try to be the salve to my father's soul, but he often treated her as the enemy, too.

Adding to my father's state of disquiet was our house's septic system. Unlike houses closer to town, out in the country we had a well for water in the backyard and two septic tanks for sewage in the front yard. For the six and a half years we spent living on Bear Tavern Road, we were on constant high alert about the septic tank. A break in the pipe between the house and one of the tanks repeatedly caused the sewage to back up into the house, overflowing out of the downstairs bathroom and sending my father into a panic of disgust.

Professionals repeatedly came to the house trying to fix the problem, including digging up the ground overlying the septic tanks to empty them and clear the lines coming to them from the house. This process led to many summer days full of the Gallagher children picking rocks out of the dirt patch on top of the septic tank to get grass to grow there again. My father either must have not wanted to spend the few dollars on topsoil or wanted to make our summers as miserable as his. When the problem came back, so did the backhoes, digging around the yard again to find the septic tank lid. And so did our duty of picking rocks out of the dirt.

Between visits by the professionals, my father would attempt to fix the problem himself. He would don his rattiest old jeans, a baggy faded-blue sweatshirt with a shredded collar and tattered cuffs, and a pair of rubber boots en route to the sump pit and sewage pipes in the basement. The dank basement was otherwise used for playing Ping-Pong or sharpening our hockey skills on the bare cement floor. When Denny went down there, though, he was all business. If we were sitting in the family room just up the stairs from where he was working, we would quickly become engulfed by the sulfurous smell and the sounds of him cursing, often calling my mother's name.

One of his trips down there became lore in our family. As he unscrewed the end of one of the sewage pipes, hoping to send a plumbing snake through the pipe to the septic tank, he was immediately drenched with all the water that had been stuck in the pipe.

"Worms!" he screamed. "Worms! Pat! Help! Worms!"

"Stay there. I'm coming!" she yelled from the kitchen.

"Worms everywhere!"

My mother ran to the basement and found my father soaked in gray water from the washing machine and showers—not the sewage from the toilets—and covered in strands of spaghetti that had gone down the kitchen sink. Years hence, we would scream, "Worms!" anytime the words *septic tank* were mentioned.

~

MY CHILDHOOD WAS PUNCTUATED WITH BEACH VACATIONS each summer, first at the Jersey Shore, often in the town of Harvey Cedars, and later via road trips to Emerald Isle, North Carolina. My father seemed happiest on vacation, particularly if we were going to the beach.

The fate of our first trip to Emerald Isle was set in New Jersey the day before we left. The chain came off my heavy steel Ross BMX bike (not quite the quality of Luke's Mongoose or the rich kids' Redlines, which I coveted), and a tooth from the chainring punctured the back of my bare heel. Being a mere ten years old, I thought nothing of it and didn't bother to tell my mother or wash the grease off. On the second night of our vacation, however, I awoke with a pain in my foot. I assumed it was early morning as there was light coming through the window. I quickly went back to sleep. When I woke up again, it was black outside.

What was happening? Had I slept through the entire day? That thought was quickly replaced with searing pain in my heel. I tried to go back to sleep, but it was no use. I sheepishly went to get my mom. I knew my father would be furious if I woke them up, but I had no choice.

"What's wrong?" my mother asked.

"My foot really hurts."

"Here, come in the bathroom with me," she whispered as she pulled the blankets off.

I followed my mother into the bathroom. She flipped on the lights and looked at my foot. "You have an infection," she said.

It was an abscess. The filthy grease injected into my heel from the chainring had created a pressurized pocket of pus below the skin of my foot with a red, tender mound surrounding it. My mother filled the bathtub with scalding hot water and put my foot in it. I howled, "It's too hot. It hurts!"

"You have to keep it in there. I will be right back."

She returned with a sewing needle and her cigarette lighter. She lit the red plastic Bic and held the flame to the business end of the needle, blackening it as it sterilized the metal. She pulled my foot out of the hot water and plunged the needle deep into my heel. I hardly felt a thing. Then she squeezed. I wailed as green pus squirted all over the bath towel my foot was on.

"Don't move."

I wiggled and squirmed. But in an instant, the pain was gone. The relief from the pressure was glorious. I returned to bed and slept like a ten-year-old should, motionless for hours.

In the morning, having survived the trauma of a needle in my foot and believing my mother was a goddam hero, I watched cartoons and ate Fruity Pebbles. My mom and dad told

Kevin and me that they were going out to look at houses and would be back in an hour. Before they left, my father offered his own brand of medical advice: "If you see a red streak going up your leg from that infection, it can go to your heart and kill you."

With that they walked out, and within minutes, Kevin and I were in tears, certain my time on this earth was limited to no more than that very day. I didn't know then that similar (though less primitive) surgical experiences would be a part of my future career.

It was common for Denny to offer these "pearls of wisdom," matter-of-fact statements filled with caveats that the world is a dangerous place, best experienced with great caution so as not to get hurt, although he allowed us to build a ten-foot-tall half-pipe made from two-by-fours and plywood in the backyard to skateboard on. His most common refrain throughout my childhood was, "Try to act normal, boys. Try to act normal."

Intermittently, my father would show flashes of joviality, but even our neighbors recognized that he was not a happy-go-lucky guy. Our most beloved neighbors were Bernie and Alice Lynch, who saw my dad and mom for exactly who they were. We lived next to the Lynches just before moving to Long Island. Bernie loved my mom tremendously. He saw the best in her. He loved us kids, too. He and Alice were like our best friends.

Mr. Lynch was in Pearl Harbor when the Japanese attacked, awakened at Hickam Field by the sounds of low-flying aircraft, then hearing the planes dropping the bombs that thrust the United States into World War II. He met Alice by accompanying her to a military dance back home in New Jersey in the middle of the war, just before being deployed again. He knew immediately that he wanted to marry her. He told her so the next day.

When he left to serve in Australia three weeks later, he wrote Alice a letter. He mailed page after page of it each day for months without ever finishing the letter. When he returned, they married, and Bernie worked as a phone repairman for the next thirty-four years. He built a modest log cabin with woods beyond the backyard, where he and Alice raised four children. As their neighbors, Kevin and I would play with their grandkids from time to time, but more often we would knock on the door and ask, "Can Mr. Lynch play?"

Mr. Lynch was my childhood hero. He was kind and patient. He was fun and funny. His stories were interesting. He rode a 1970s Honda motorcycle at age fifty-six when we moved in. He and Alice seemed to age backward, looking younger at sixty-six than they did at fifty-six. For our tenth birthday, Mr. Lynch took Kevin and me each for a ride on his motorcycle, equipped with a windscreen and bright yellow gas tank. It was the thrill of our lives at the time.

Later in life, when I graduated medical school, Mr. Lynch told me, "You two showed absolutely no signs of intelligence as kids. The two of you would stand back-to-back raking leaves and hit each other in the head with the rake handles. I had to separate you every time. And you'd ask for hot chocolate after two minutes."

It was the best compliment he could have ever given me. He passed away after he fractured his hip while I was in my surgical residency—an injury I would go on to treat thousands of and see firsthand the toll it can take on an elderly person. Alice followed a few years later. I still miss Bernie and Alice every day.

In high school, I began to care less about school and more about partying. I spent time hanging out with friends as far away from Denny as I could get. At the end of tenth grade, I came down with a severe case of mononucleosis. I missed the last three weeks of school, including all my final exams. The academic repercussions didn't faze me. Missing out on seeing my friends did. The doctors had warned my mother not to let me go to school or go out at all. It was the sickest I had felt in my life, including a bout of pneumonia at age seven that kept me at home for two weeks. Going up the stairs was exhausting. I recall stopping to sit and rest at the top of our short staircase from the foyer to the second floor because my legs felt impossibly heavy. I slept a ton.

At the end of my sophomore year, my father's company offered him a chance to run a penicillin plant in Smithfield, North Carolina, far away from his boss. My dad jumped at the opportunity. We moved to the northern part of Raleigh just before my sixteenth birthday.

Dad seemed genuinely happy when we got there. My mom had a different experience. Though she didn't mind moving to a new state with a completely different culture, her relationship with Denny seemed to worsen, making her feel isolated. She wanted to move back to New Jersey.

My brother and I finished the last two years of high school at a place called Ravenscroft. It was a small private school with just over fifty students per grade, many of whom had been there since they were five years old. Within the first week, Kevin and I made friends with a kid named Vincent Taylor.

"This really excited kid came up to me and started pointing at me and saying, 'You changed clothes!'" I told Kevin at the end of school one day during our first week.

"That's Vincent Taylor," Kevin offered.

"He seems hilarious," I replied.

Vincent lived on a beautiful farm in a small town called Archer Lodge an hour east of our house, about forty-five minutes from school. His mother had moved out there after his parents' divorce back in elementary school. Vincent had been at Ravenscroft since kindergarten, but he was not like most of the other students—wealthy and well-mannered southern preppies, several of whom drove brand-new sports cars bequeathed to them by their parents on their sixteenth birthdays. Vincent drove a BMW, but it had faded, blotchy paint like an old tattoo and windows he tinted so dark that light barely made it through to the back seats. The car had been abandoned for years in one of his barns, collecting dust, spiderwebs, and acorns from the squirrels. Vincent fixed up the two-door 3 Series and had it running in time to get his driver's license. He could repair just about anything.

Out at his farm he would ride wheelies on his four-wheeler, take us swimming and fishing in his pond, and go off-roading in his 1965 International Scout—a vehicle also left for dead a decade or so earlier after the ocean's tide had washed up over it on the beach. We had never met anyone like him.

Vincent was in everyone's good graces, from parents to teachers to girls to the local merchants. We would go to the C.E. Barnes Store, where Vincent would fill up his BMW's gas tank, get a few Pepsis and some pork rinds—a delicacy we didn't have where I was from in New Jersey—then head for the counter. An older gentleman sat behind the cash register, smoking a cigarette and watching TV. He was dressed in worn denim jeans and a plaid shirt with mother-of-pearl snaps.

"How are y'all doing today, Vincent?" he would ask.

"Doing great, Mr. Barnes. Just raisin' hell, as usual."

Mr. Barnes pulled out a small billing pad and wrote down Vincent's purchases.

"Sign here, Vincent," he'd say in his gravelly, slow southern way.

In lieu of his signature, Vincent would draw pictures of his mom's house along with a few horses and pigs. Mr. Barnes just chuckled.

For growing up in such a rural area in North Carolina, Vincent spoke without a trace of a southern drawl. His friends out at the farm spoke with thick accents and dressed differently than we did in the suburbs. Most of them cropped tobacco in the summer and drove pickup trucks with Confederate flags adorning them.

Vincent's closest neighbor was a Black man named Samuel who lived with his family in a tiny, one-story house along the dirt road running through the field by Vincent's biggest barn. The house had no running water. I'm not sure it even had electricity. Samuel worked for one man in town with an unwritten understanding that he would not work for anyone else without permission. It was as close to modern-day indentured servitude as possible.

Samuel was granted permission to work for Vincent's mom whenever she needed him out on the farm, adding on an enclosed porch to her kitchen, building fences, and repairing the decades-old tobacco barns. Samuel's accent was one that I simply could not understand; it was as if he was speaking a different language. I'd stare at Vincent in disbelief as he easily conversed with Samuel.

Life with Vincent was never dull. We would visit his dad's house in Raleigh, where the front hall closet was shaped like an ear and the back porch towered thirty feet above the ground without any railing. His father sold a company that designed one of the first barcode readers and spent most of his time tinkering around in his shop, designing boats with experimental hulls or any other number of toys. In the kitchen, Mr. Taylor built a fish tank that hung down from the ceiling like *La Pyramide Inversée* at the Louvre in Paris. I could see where Vincent got his creativity and mechanical mind.

Mr. Taylor had remarried a woman who sported resting bitch face before it was even a thing. Vincent didn't care much for her, and neither did we. So on Wednesdays when Vincent was supposed to sleep at his father's house, he often slept on the couch in our family room instead.

With Vincent and a few other friends from Ravenscroft, we would drive around Raleigh and the surrounding towns, barely escaping trouble. One weekend we went to a junkyard out in the country to steal parts from cars. Another weekend, we climbed on the roof of a local grocery store, drinking beer and kicking the gravel rocks that would spark and luminesce as they struck each other. We canoed in the Falls of the Neuse River, drove the BMW down dirt roads and over jumps, and parked at the airport to watch the planes land.

Our group included an eclectic cadre of friends. Alison was a senior, with a set of auspicious breasts that drove all the guys crazy. She was hilarious and unassuming. We helped her with her math homework while she managed to entertain us and laugh at our jokes. Charlie was the starting quarterback and homecoming king who sidled into our group just as his parents went through a terrible divorce. Charlie lived at our house for the final three months of high school as his home life imploded. Rod was the youngest child of an older, wealthy father who remarried when the children from his first marriage were adults. Rod's parents treated us like kings. Their seven-thousand-square-foot house left plenty of room for us to drink beer, watch movies, and play video games in Rod's wing of the mansion without being disturbed.

Denny became more relaxed in North Carolina when it came to parenting. He loved Alison and Vincent, and we seemed to get away with just about anything when we were with them. He still showed his temper periodically and seemed to take more of it out on my mom than he had before. Still, he suggested to me that I wasn't cut out for college and offered to give Kevin one of the cars if he wanted to move out and never come back. There was never a dull moment with Denny, either.

Even with our crew in North Carolina, Kevin and I missed our friends from New Jersey. Luke was still in Pennington, and Liam was in boarding school in Delaware. Liam's parents had moved to Maryland at the same time we moved to North Carolina, so we decided we would all get back together there for a weekend.

Kevin and I drove up and met Liam and Luke at Liam's house. The four of us left the following day to go see the Grateful Dead in Landover, Maryland. Not having planned very far in advance, we spent several hours in the stadium parking lot looking for tickets, but there were none to be found. At some point, we encountered a friendly guy in green corduroy Ocean Pacific shorts sitting on a grassy hill at the edge of the parking lot. We asked him if he had any tickets for the show.

"Right on, right on. No. Sorry, brothers."

"Thanks, anyway."

"Right on. I do have some kind bud, though, if you're looking to buy some," he added.

We looked at each other, confused and thinking he was saying "time bud," not knowing what either *kind bud* or *time bud* were. We played along as if we knew what he was talking about and declined his offer. As he continued his sales pitch, he lay back against the hill with his legs spread until his testicles appeared from under the bottom of his shorts. We could barely contain our laughter as we glanced dartingly from each other down to his balls and back to each other. After giving it a little more thought and laughing at the ridiculous situation, we bought a bag of the pot he was peddling and headed back to the car.

By late afternoon we realized there was no way we were getting into the concert given the scarcity of tickets. Luke, Liam, and I decided it was time to try the kind bud. We were going to be in the parking lot until after the concert let out, and hopefully this would be a fun way to pass the time. Kevin, who had always been more reluctant to try drugs than I was, opted for drinking beer instead.

As the sun went down, we walked around, taking in the freak show that is a Grateful Dead parking lot scene. There seemed to be as many people outside as there must have been inside the stadium. Smoking the kind bud led to a high unlike anything I had ever experienced before. There were no hallucinations, but the flashing lights and glowing Frisbees almost seemed alive. We imagined we were having as much fun in the parking lot as we would have at the concert.

The peaceful, festive vibe of the parking lot came to a screeching halt for a few minutes when an agitated high schooler, seemingly fucked up on LSD or something similar, started screaming and making a huge scene. He stumbled across the parking lot, bouncing off one person and then another until he knocked over a pristine vintage Indian motorcycle and dented the gas tank. The jubilant crowd fell silent. The intoxicated kid lay half on the ground, half on a wheel of the once-beautiful motorcycle, legs akimbo. The owner of the bike, a massive, bearded man standing nearby, looked at his bike and then at the grunting kid. Friends of the kid quickly dragged him away as best they could.

"What the fuck!" said the Goliath, picking up his Indian and rubbing his forehead in disbelief. "I should have beat the shit out of that kid."

As the crowd slowly resumed its revelry, we listened to the faint sounds of the concert, trying to decipher what song the band was playing. At 11:00 p.m., we packed up our stuff and sped north on the highway toward Liam's house, with Kevin behind the wheel. Nearly immediately I began to feel carsick. Twenty minutes into the ride, I said, "I'm going to throw up."

"Okay, I'll pull over," Kevin said.

I couldn't wait, though. So as we continued driving at highway speed, I opened the door and started vomiting, not caring or sensing that I wasn't wearing a seatbelt. Luke quickly put his index finger around my belt loop. "Don't worry, I've got him," he said. I vomited two more times then closed the door and slumped over.

Kevin pulled off the highway at the next exit, drove immediately into a neighborhood, and stopped. I got out of the car and crawled onto the lawn of the house we were parked in front of. Thankfully the vomiting was over, so I cleaned my filthy hands on the dewy grass as the boys stared at me in pity. I lay there for a few minutes, then gargled some water and got back in the car, riding the rest of the way to Liam's house in silence. We pulled into the driveway, and the four of us staggered up to the front door. It was locked. We didn't have a key. As Liam rang the doorbell, I had a terrible feeling. His father opened the door in his bathrobe.

"Hi, Dad," Liam said, then paused. "Did you feed the cat?"

"You guys look terrible. Go to bed," his dad replied in his proper British accent, then turned and walked upstairs.

We bounced off each other as we all tried to get in the front door at the same time, then we lumbered up the stairs. As we all lay down in sleeping bags on the floor of Liam's room, my head continued to spin. I was not having fun anymore.

"If I wake up and I'm still high, I am going to kill myself," I stated emphatically.

When the light of day woke me in the morning, I was incredibly thankful to feel sober and be thinking clearly. The four of us who had been best friends since before elementary school laid around, recounting the wild events of the prior night then of the past fifteen years. To avoid Liam's parents, we headed stealthily down the stairs and straight out the front door to find breakfast in the form of bagels and coffee. As we got in the car, I reached to close the door in the back seat, and my fingers gripped the remaining chunks of vomit still clinging to the handle. I wanted to throw up again. The boys gagged as I flung the disgusting emesis to the ground with the flip of my wrist. What a trip.

BACK IN NORTH CAROLINA, KEVIN AND I WOULD FORM A bond with Vincent that would last a lifetime. The following year another new student, Jon Cranford, joined the school. Refusing to go by his first name, he preferred to be called Cranford, though some called him Flash, a tease about his lack of acceleration on the sports fields.

Cranford started almost every sentence by saying, "Dude, man, dude," and would greet girls and guys alike with a singsong "Heyyyy, duuuude," that would become his calling card. We loved him immediately. His mumbling was at times as hard to understand as Vincent's neighbor Samuel, but that added to his charm. He had braces that stayed on his teeth for nearly all of high school and college. At any given moment there were bright orange bits of ToastChee Sandwich Crackers accumulated in the corners of his mouth and between the metal brackets of his braces. He drank Coke from sunup to sundown and chain-smoked Marlboros. He loved to tell stories of his years at boarding school in the Northeast and ask everyone about the details of their lives. He had as much character as anyone at Ravenscroft.

As a twin, all my friendships to that point in my life were ones that I shared with Kevin: Luke, Liam, Vincent, Alison, Cranford. The relationship with an identical twin is unlike any other. Identical twins share the same genetic code and as such respond in very similar ways to the world. An exception to this is a less common form of identical twins called *mirror twins* in which the fertilized egg splits at a slightly later date and the twins are essentially mirror images of each other. Often one of these twins is left-handed while the other is right. Birthmarks or freckles are on the left for one twin and the right for the other. One twin may be more analytical while the other is more artistic. Kevin and I are the more common type of identical twins and are incredibly alike.

My mother expected a child to be born in August of 1972, but she did not expect to have two of them. It was not until after her first son was born, slated to be named Kevin Michael Gallagher, that the doctor told her she was having twins. At that time, ultrasound use was not widespread, and my mother's doctor did not perform one. Obstetricians simply listened for the baby's heartbeat and asked expecting mothers about the baby's movements. More than one fetal heartbeat and the mother was expecting twins. In the case of my mother, the doctor missed the second heartbeat, Kevin's or mine. Either our hearts were in perfect synchrony, or he thought he was hearing one fetal heartbeat and one maternal heartbeat. My mother soon learned of his mistake.

"This isn't over. There is another foot," the doctor told my mother as she lay recovering from just giving birth to my brother.

"What?" she exclaimed.

"You're having twins!"

Nine minutes later I was born. Kevin Michael Gallagher had turned into Kevin *and* Michael Gallagher. Kevin was born both first and headfirst, whereas I came out breech afterward. As infants, we looked so much alike, though, that my mother likely mixed us up at some point, not knowing which one of us was the first to be born. Because we were so similar, our mother kept our hospital bracelets on to tell us apart until our wrists were too fat to safely do so. Perhaps a tattoo may have been a more reliable method.

The similarities didn't end there. We grew up being dressed alike by our mother for the first five years or so, as many twins do. These days, when I look at baby pictures, I cannot tell us apart. I even get confused at some pictures of us after the age of ten. Listening to our voices on a tape recorder as a kid, I heard only Kevin's voice — same intonations, same pronunciations, same cadences. We were physical and intellectual equals. For years we got the same grades, ran the same speed, jumped just as high as one another. Life events eventually started to shape our personalities in different ways, though, as the years went on. Watching something the other didn't on TV or reading a different book would influence one and not the other. Getting caught and yelled at for doing something mischievous caused angst that only one felt.

By high school we were still very similar but no longer identical in our behaviors. I was a more serious student; Kevin was more outgoing and social. We fought increasingly over fatuous stuff. I was sick of being by his side. He may have felt the same about me. We applied to different colleges. I was sure I would get into the University of Colorado Boulder. He applied to Colorado State University and hoped his SATs would get him in because his grades certainly would not. I was overconfident and got waitlisted at CU, then rejected. Kevin was accepted to CSU with contingencies. I announced I would go anywhere to college except to school with Kevin. He made no such declaration.

After just a year apart, I missed Kevin and decided we were better off in college together. So I transferred to CSU, where we would again share a house, a group of close friends, and experiences that far exceeded my drugged-out night at the Grateful Dead concert.

Chapter 2

The Shake

In college I began to bike and run to feel more alive. Sitting and studying was getting to me, and running was a good way to burn off some steam or cure a Saturday morning hangover. As a kid I was moderately athletic, but never excelled in any one sport. I played hockey for many years in New Jersey along with other typical kids' sports, like soccer, swimming, and baseball. I was a terrible soccer player and a decent swimmer. My brother and I were both pretty good at hitting a baseball but not that great at fielding. At Ravenscroft, I played lacrosse for a couple of years and enjoyed it without a ton of prowess, but Vincent and Cranford were on the team, too, so it was fun. I would run occasionally to get in shape for hockey or lacrosse season, but I was by no means a runner in the true sense. I thought the kids who ran cross-country were nuts for running as far and as often as they did. Besides, they were way too fast for me to keep up with. Even as a little kid, I would bike five miles with Kevin to the pool in the summer, but neither of us ever went out bicycling specifically for exercise.

When I moved to Colorado for my sophomore year of college, I fell in love with the beauty of the Rocky Mountains. I immediately bought a mountain bike and rode it just about everywhere. It was my sole source of transportation, and my way of getting into the mountains easily. We lived just three blocks east of the Colorado State University campus in Fort Collins, Colorado. Six of us shared a five-bedroom house. I was a late addition to the mix, transferring from North Carolina State University after my freshman year.

NC State simply was not my cup of tea. The campus was a never-ending parade of brick buildings on top of brick quads with powerlines running every which way overhead and lots of conservative southern culture. Still, the school was good for me academically. I was in the engineering program, and classes like calculus and Fortran were both challenging and stimulating. I immediately raised my academic game and began studying like mad to keep up. It paid off my second semester when I made the dean's list. After receiving my grades and going home to New Jersey, where my parents had since moved back to, I came to realize that I did not need to be stuck somewhere that made me unhappy. No one was forcing me to stay at NC State. I was an adult capable of making my own decisions regarding my present and future career and happiness. It was an epiphany.

When I visited Kevin at Colorado State University, the students there just seemed more cheerful and in line with my views of the world. Plus, Vincent was just an hour away at CU Boulder. CSU was not the best academic school I was capable of transferring to, but it had other things I wanted. I considered CU Boulder, but I didn't apply because I wanted an environmental engineering degree or something similar. I may have felt slighted about my prior rejection from CU, as well, or worried I might be rebuffed yet again. So I applied to transfer to CSU in June, got accepted in July, and left for Colorado in August. Before I departed New Jersey, I called my girlfriend at NC State and told her I'd never be coming back. That was the last time we ever spoke.

It was the best decision of my life.

My academic career at CSU took an inauspicious turn just a few weeks after arriving. Loaded up on science classes for my new major, environmental health, I was preparing for my first exam in my room on a Sunday afternoon. This exam would set the tone for my future at this new college and hopefully be a continuation of the great grades I had achieved at NC State.

On a quick break, I went upstairs to hang out with my roommates in the spacious living room of our 1910 brick bungalow. As I sat with them on our dusty couches, an attractive, thin college-aged girl appeared at our glass-paned front door and began to knock. One of us answered it, and she smiled and told us that her name was Athena. She was a Stanford student en route to California and had come to town to see her boyfriend, who lived just a few doors down.

"I was supposed to stay with him, but he says he doesn't want me there," she explained with a slightly exasperated expression on her face.

This all-too-trusting, or perhaps desperate, woman had seen us out in the front yard earlier in the day and decided we were her best option for a place to crash. As we sat around the living room and talked, Athena's magnetism and intelligence seemed to appeal to each of us.

"I have some acid if anyone wants to take it with me," she said, clearly referring to LSD, a drug I had always been wary of.

"I am in the middle of studying for an exam," I said without hesitation, "but thanks for the offer."

I returned to my room and buried my head in the books once again. By 10:00 p.m., exhausted from studying, I was feeling both prepared for my first exam at CSU and ready for bed. I sauntered up the back stairs from my makeshift basement bedroom to say goodnight and make a plea for the rest of the household to respect my need for sleep, asking them to keep it to a dull roar for the evening. I took a moment to drink a single beer, and then in a moment of unusual capriciousness, said, "Fuck it." I told Athena I would take the LSD with her. We stayed up for hours talking the way only college kids with no real worries can do and laughing the way only people on acid can. After nearly seven hours of talking without pretext about life and love and the stars, I went to bed just past 5:00 a.m., setting my alarm to get up in time to study for an hour or two before my 11:00 a.m. exam.

The next moment of awareness I had was my friend Brian shaking me and telling me to get up as my alarm blared.

"Where am I?" I mumbled.

I had been sleeping through the loud beeping for nearly two hours and had precious little time to shower and get to campus before my test. I sprinted up the stairs, out the door, and onto my bike, beelining to school while still woozy from drugs and lack of sleep. What the hell was I thinking? This was my first exam in a required biology course that I could not fail. This was the type of stupid shit other people did, not me. I gathered my composure and read the exam questions, trying to focus. I plodded my way through it, at times stopping to chastise myself. I went home that day full of worry that I had made a mistake transferring to CSU, thinking I had blown my chance to start out on the right foot.

Three days later, I learned that I got an A on the exam, thanking my lucky stars that no damage had been done to my academic career. It spooked me a skosh, but not enough to slow down my social life. There was still a lot of fun to be had in Fort Collins, a town at the forefront of the microbrew revolution about to take place in America.

Mountain biking was at the top of my priority list beyond school and partying. I bought a white hardtail Mongoose bike (a lingering desire from my childhood) and put a state-of-the-art Manitou front shock on it. I began to ride the five miles from our house out to the foothills surrounding Horsetooth Reservoir as much as I could, always dressed in purple cotton Gramicci shorts, Saucony sneakers, and whatever cotton concert or local beer T-shirt I had on that day. Early on, the altitude and the cigarettes I smoked periodically made for a tough slog. So I kicked the cigs habit and before I knew it, I was riding up the steep gravel road with ease, then down the local favorite A Trail. The technical, rocky terrain took a heavy toll on the frame's white paint as I went ass over teakettle, flying above the handlebars with every bump. I learned quickly what the cacti of Colorado look and feel like to bare skin and how rocky the Rocky Mountains truly are. It became a daily routine for me in the spring of my first year there.

I finished my first semester with decent grades and having had a lot of fun. My wavy hair grew long, I dated a pretty, fit blonde girl from my chemistry class, and I made a handful of new friends. Spring semester seemed to go equally as well, but organic chemistry was a thorn in my side, not unlike the cacti I had encountered biking. I preferred math and physics to chemistry, which seemed nebulous to me at times.

Before my organic chemistry final exam that May, the class average was a dismal 45 percent. A grade of 66 percent allowed any student to be exempt from the final and receive an A for the semester. I was barely clinging to a C+ based on the curve. Studying for the final was maddening. I simply wasn't understanding the material the way I needed to. I resorted to memorizing the study guide that was handed out the last week of class and ignored the rest of the material from the semester. When that became overwhelming on the day of the exam, I set out on my bike for Horsetooth. It was a far better option than taking LSD. The ride seemed to clear my head, and I got back just in time for the test, which looked remarkably similar to the study guide. *You lucky bastard*, I thought to myself. I aced the test and finished with a B in the class, leaving me with only one chemistry class and lab left in my college career. I couldn't have been happier. I discovered the real power that exercise had on my cognitive ability along with the notion that luck favors the prepared!

From that point on, I started using exercise to sharpen my mental focus. I wasn't done dabbling in drugs to expand my mind in other ways, but running and biking were far more interesting. From the time the trails were cleared of ice in the spring until the snow started falling in November, I traded my Saucony running shoes for my new Italian Sidi Dominator mountain bike shoes and my Mongoose for a mint-green Specialized Stumpjumper that was as pretty to look at as it was fun to ride. I had come a long way since my Ross BMX bike. I explored Lory State Park, Hewlett Gulch, Boulder's Walker Ranch, and Golden's White Ranch. I sizzled with excitement each time I went for a new ride.

NEARLY FIFTEEN MONTHS AFTER GETTING TO CSU, WITH A full year of classes behind me and an increasingly difficult course load, I felt settled in. My studies were important to me, and I often wondered if I would stay in the field of environmental health, or if I would consider medical school. That year, I dated a girl whose mother was an emergency physician back in Cincinnati. The romantic notion of being a doctor appealed to me, and my girlfriend encouraged me to consider it. Besides, the sciences were my forte, and I was taking every class required for entry to medical school just by getting my degree in environmental health.

When I wasn't studying, I was wrapped up in skiing and running and biking, either with friends or by myself. I didn't mind being alone when I was enjoying the outdoors. There was still plenty of time to socialize at night. We hosted tons of parties at our house, and our circle of friends seemed to grow and grow. I had nerdy friends from my science classes, many of whom were trying to get into the renowned veterinary school at CSU. I had hippie friends who went to see Phish and Widespread Panic concerts with Kevin and me. I had running and biking friends, too. These were often totally separate worlds, and only the rarest of friends fit into all three groups. In some ways I wondered which of those three I really was, and in other ways I was confident that I was all of them. I enjoyed that my brother and I were known on campus as the really smart twins even with our shoulder-length hair and Earth Day T-shirts.

My wild side still was capable of getting the best of me, though. Kevin and Vincent and I would go out to the bars and get hammered drinking Odell 90 Shilling Ale or New Belgium Fat Tire with whatever poor souls we brought along on any given night. We rode our bikes around town shit-faced, and many fell victim to our antics. Vincent's girlfriend got her front wheel stuck in the railroad tracks on Mulberry Street and went over the bars, face-planting onto the road. She arose from the pavement holding her chin. "Which way is the hospital?" Two hours later she was all patched up with a set of stitches in her face, courtesy of Poudre Valley Hospital.

That same summer, Vincent's roommate, Dave, hit a cement light pole while biking back to our house after a party. As he lay unconscious on the ground with agonal breathing—the gasping type people experience before dying—Vincent cackled, pointing at him and yelling, "He's snorting!" Yet another trip to Poudre Valley Hospital.

As Kevin, Vincent, and Dave rode around campus that night before the hospital visit, I tried to beat them home by taking a shortcut through campus. As I sped along between the massive edifices of the student center and the library, I suddenly struck a metal bar at chest level, not aware I was headed straight toward a standing bike rack. I was thrown violently backward off my bike as though Hulk Hogan had just clotheslined me in the ring. As I lay on the ground, two students appeared, standing over me and asking if I was okay.

"I think I'm fine," I reassured them, not fully knowing if that was true. I barely felt a thing in my inebriated state.

Dave was not as lucky as I was. He awoke the next morning in a sling with dried blood crusted in his ear and streaked down his cheek—a broken collarbone and a ruptured eardrum.

There were plenty of other non-bike-related incidents, too. Vincent split his tongue in half as we skied out of bounds on Loveland Pass over the so-called Ironing Board, striking his chin on his knee as he compressed on the flat landing. He offered to drive himself to the hospital being as familiar with it as he was. Our friend Davis crashed into a curb and shattered his eye socket, nearly mangling his face for life and ultimately sending him to the operating room at Poudre Valley Hospital. His roommate broke both of his tibiae while skiing over a cliff out of bounds and lay in the cold for hours until the search and rescue could come get him. Drugs and alcohol were a common thread through a lot of these stories. How we all made it out alive is a mystery.

The apogee of this type of behavior came at the start of my fourth semester at CSU. A couple of my roommates decided that they would buy a quarter-pounder. Not a hamburger from McDonald's, mind you, but a quarter pound of psilocybin mushrooms. After Kevin carefully weighed it out into quarter-ounce baggies to dole out to our wide circle of friends, there was nothing but dust and crumbs left at the bottom of the gallon storage bag—the shake. Not wanting anything to go to waste, Kevin offered up the remainder for anyone to take. It had been a while since I'd done any drugs, and I figured what the hell. Not knowing that the shake was the most powerful part of what that quarter-pound bag had to offer, we finished off everything that remained.

As we sat in my brother's bedroom waiting for the entertaining effects of the mushrooms to commence, we sipped on local IPAs and bullshitted with each other, telling jokes and stories, recalling the close calls and hospital visits we'd had over the years. Then, like the flicker when a villain interrupts a nation's pleasant TV broadcast in a movie, I started having sudden, staticky hallucinations that I was outdoors. The faces of my brother and my roommates became rocky outcroppings of imaginary mountainsides. The walls rapidly expanded and closed back in with each breath. I had taken mushrooms and acid before, but never had hallucinations like this.

Kevin repeatedly felt his pants and shirt, asking, "Why am I all wet?" He was perfectly dry. Our roommate Keith began to laugh hysterically like some sort of mad joker, his face turning beet red. Another roommate, Skip, retreated to his bedroom, where he hallucinated that the fishes from the tank in the living room were swimming out of the glass, through his slightly ajar door, around his room, and back into the tank.

The shake was unleashing its mighty power on us without restraint.

What was fun at first for me soon became very unpleasant. I lay down in my bed and began to imagine awful images. I got a paper bag and leaned over the side of my futon and vomited. I saw the faces of monsters with jagged teeth coming from triangular jaws emerging from the emesis toward me. It was not the night I was hoping for. I went to my dingy basement bathroom and showered, hoping to sober up. No such luck.

After looking in the mirror above the bathroom sink and seeing my face severely distorted, I went back to my room and scribbled a note: "I walked to the hospital. Don't worry, I'm okay."

So up the stairs and out the back door I went. Only one step outside into the frigid night air, and I immediately slipped on the ice, landing hard on the ground. Pain! A familiar sensation. *Okay*, I thought. *I'm okay. I felt that. That's normal. I'm going to get through this.*

When we are in trouble or in times of desperation, we all need something familiar, something reassuring. For me that night, pain was the only thing remotely recognizable as such.

I walked around to the front of the house and out into the street. I took a right, then half a block later I got confused as to where I was. Which way was the hospital? Did I even know how to get there? Was I still close to my house? We had been to Poudre Valley Hospital so many times, and now I couldn't find my way there.

Lights were on in the house I stood in front of, where a group of people slightly older than me socialized inside. I walked up to the door and knocked. A man in his mid-twenties with curly hair and groovy clothes answered. He seemed to recognize me, though no one else there did. Did I know him? Was this the neighbor we referred to as "Stuck in the Seventies Eddie"? I'd only seen him from afar before.

I opened my mouth and the following words flowed out: "Hi. I'm Michael. I'm on mushrooms. Can someone here take me to the hospital?"

The group of men and women burst out laughing. They couldn't control themselves. I stood there saying nothing. Tripping balls.

Eddie said, "Let me take you upstairs to my room."

"Okay."

I walked into the house and past all the partygoers, who were giggling and staring at me as I went by. The steep staircase in the back of the house led us up to Eddie's small room with low, vaulted ceilings. I remained in my heavy winter jacket and sat on the floor. Eddie asked me what I had taken and when.

I said, "I think I might throw up, again."

"Again?"

"Yeah," I croaked.

Eddie departed and quickly returned with a pot for me to vomit in if the need arose. He reassured me that the hospital was not the best place for me and that he would take care of me. I asked him if he had any medicine to make me sleepy, and he said, "No way, man." He made awkward small talk with me for the next hour or two while I hallucinated and ruminated, fidgeting the whole time.

Then suddenly, with what seemed like a vacuum sucking the hallucinations out of me, I stopped seeing the unreal, snapped out of my delirium, and became immediately, fantastically sober. I told him I was feeling better and that I now knew where I was. I would just walk home. He walked me downstairs, past those I'd entertained with my grand entrance, and out the front door. He blithely waved goodbye and watched me walk the half block home.

I walked up the front steps out of the cold night air and into our warm house. It was close to midnight. I opened the door and casually took a seat with everybody. No one had realized I was gone. I told them what had happened, and they laughed as hard as Eddie's friends. I was so fucking happy to no longer be hallucinating that it felt euphoric, and I couldn't have cared less who was laughing. I stayed up for hours just enjoying my rational thoughts. That was the last time I ever did illicit drugs.

From that point on, I made academics my priority. I still had fun, but never at the expense of my education. My grades improved from there, and I started to consider medical school more seriously. I would graduate on time with a great GPA and a job doing environmental health and occupational safety at Poudre Valley Hospital, of all places. Perhaps they appreciated all the business we gave them, though not from me that night on psychedelics.

Before graduating, I contemplated my future academic life and career. Medical school was still a pipe dream at that point. I had the grades and all the prerequisites, but I still hadn't tackled the MCAT entrance exams—a test that requires months of preparation, the score of which seals the fate of each applicant's chances for entry to medical school. I could see myself as a doctor, but a decade more of schooling and training seemed too daunting. Instead of the MCATs, I took the GRE test for graduate school. With minimal prep, I crushed it and then applied to several schools of public health. I was accepted to the PhD program at the University of North Carolina Gillings School of Global Public Health. I would follow in the footsteps of my eldest sister, Kelly, who was an undergraduate in Chapel Hill in the 1980s, and my other sister, Kristi, who had a master's degree from the school of public health there. Kristi was still living in Chapel Hill with her husband, Andrew. It seemed like a perfect fit. To boot, I was given a full scholarship along with a stipend for living expenses.

While working at Poudre Valley Hospital, however, I decided I would not be satisfied unless I took the MCATs. Even though I had been accepted to the school of public health, there was something I really liked about working in a hospital, and I grew more in love with the idea of being a doctor. Books like *The Cider House Rules* made me think I might be a rural country doctor or an obstetrician. Being a surgeon wasn't really on my radar, although I had always had a knack for working with my hands doing woodworking and carpentry.

Months after finishing up at CSU, I fell in love with a girl I'd known from college. She had disappeared for a year while studying abroad in Ireland, then reappeared just as I graduated. For as long as I'd known Fiona, she had dated a guy named Calvin. I don't think I'd ever met Calvin, but I knew he lived up in the mountains, and I pictured a lumberjack when I thought of him. Fiona and Calvin had broken up while she was in Ireland. She was single and so was I. We saw each other one evening at a bar in town, and before I knew it, we were dating, then living together with two other female roommates in a spacious basement apartment.

Living with a woman for the first time was exciting. I enjoyed the closeness to Fiona that came along with it. I would work days at the hospital, and Fiona would work evenings at a new bar in town, taking classes during the day to finish her degree. I would go sit at the bar and read books while she served drinks and waited tables. Most of my college buddies had moved elsewhere, so my social life revolved nearly exclusively around Fiona. She was my closest friend.

Then one day, things changed. Calvin fell off the roof of a house while working and sustained a traumatic brain injury. He spent the next several months in a Denver hospital convalescing. Fiona heard the news and went to see him right away. The shock of his condition must have changed her feelings for him. She began to talk about Calvin constantly and called me his name repeatedly. I was young and not particularly jealous of a guy who was incapacitated in the hospital, but I could tell our relationship was different. We would grow apart as a result of her new involvement with Calvin's health. I told her I was going to Chapel Hill by myself, not even asking what her plans were. It was painful, and I look back on it without fond memories. It would shape the way I dealt with the illness of one of my wife's friends in the future.

The sting of this relationship disaster was soon eased with a trip to Europe with Kevin and our good friend, Ryan, a fun-loving kid we met through Vincent. Kevin was about to start a master's program in economics at Tufts as I was about to start graduate school, so this was a perfect way to spend our last month together. We begged Vincent to come with us, but he insisted there was kayaking to do, though we found out later his decision was based on a girl.

The three of us made our way to New Jersey, stayed with the Phillipses in Pennington for a night, and then departed for Europe from Philadelphia—the first time I'd ever be using my passport. We landed at Heathrow amidst a record heat wave, learning that ice was a rare commodity in Europe in those days. We spent the next month staying in youth hostels, riding trains, and carrying backpacks around the likes of London, Amsterdam, and Prague, meeting tons of interesting and friendly people along the way. Some mistook us for band members because of our long hair, a common misunderstanding when all my friends and I traveled together. I went off by myself for a few days to Ireland, where I stayed with friends Fiona had made when she was in school in Dublin. It was a treat, but it was hard to explain to her friends my feelings for her and the complexity Calvin's injury added to our relationship.

Ryan and Kevin were great company. Ryan was easy to travel with and kept us entertained by constantly delivering sardonic one-liners. Despite his snark, he was one of the kindest souls we knew. He grew up in Southern California and then came to Colorado for college. His dad, Ron, migrated to Colorado soon after Ryan did. He owned a business just outside Boulder called Backpacker's Pantry that sold packaged, freeze-dried food in stores like REI. Ron was a shrewd businessman and a great dad. He made friends with us and treated us like family.

When we returned from Europe, Kevin headed for Boston, I for Chapel Hill, and Ryan back to Nederland, a town in the foothills of Colorado about twenty miles up Boulder Canyon.

Ned, as it is known, fit Ryan well. It was quiet but with a crunchy, funky feel.

When I got to Chapel Hill, I socialized with the other students in the school of public health, but they never felt like the group of friends I had in college. I started to wonder if I just had a tough time making friends. I had a girlfriend my freshman year without Kevin, but not a group of guys I liked hanging out with. The same had happened the year after college and now again in graduate school. Thankfully, I had a great roommate, Nici, a woman from Germany in a foreign exchange program whose English was better than most Americans I knew. We rarely went out together, but she was great company in our two-bedroom house and kept me from getting lonely.

One day a few of the women from my public health program asked me to join them for a long run as part of their training for the annual Marine Corps Marathon. I told them I didn't run marathons, but would love to tag along. I met them that Saturday on Franklin Street at the edge of campus, and we headed out for our jog together. The pace was slower than I was used to, but I was happy to be out for a run with other people. We chitchatted the miles away and before I knew it, I had run thirteen miles with them—the longest run I had ever completed. *Well, shit, that was easy*, I thought. *If I just slow down a little, I can probably run even farther.* So the next week I joined them again, and they convinced me to run the marathon with them. Registration was not online at the time, so I simply showed up with cash to pay for an entry the day before the race.

The race itself was huge, unlike anything I'd ever seen. It took more than fifteen minutes for everyone to get across the start line after the gun went off. Despite the huge differential, we were all given the same start time, unlike today's methods using chip time like at the Pocono Marathon. My friends and I weaved in and out of a heavy crowd of runners until we found a cohesive group running about the same pace we intended to go. Two of the women from Chapel Hill and I tried to keep up with each other for a while, but eventually we splintered apart.

It grew warm during the race, and my cotton Cal Berkeley T-shirt dampened with sweat and began to chafe the skin at the back of my armpits. My nutrition plan that included eating gels—small packets that contain simple sugars for quick energy—that I had finagled over our long training runs was intact until mile eighteen, when I was handed a peanut butter and chocolate energy bar. My resolve to stick to my plan was weakened by my hunger and fatigue, so I decided to try it. What a rookie mistake it turned out to be. The bar congealed into a thick, sticky ball of glue in my mouth. I could barely swallow it and was forced to spit most of it out. Worse, it made my mouth intensely dry, coating my tongue and the roof of my mouth with a sugary film. I was

desperate for a drink of water, which I wouldn't find for
another mile.

I quickly grew increasingly tired until I began to alternate
between walking and running. What had happened? I'd run
twenty miles in training, and here I was at mile twenty-one at
risk of not finishing. Determined not to surrender, I kept
moving. Each mile seemed to have no end. Eventually I
sensed the finish line was close enough to make it the rest of
the way without walking, and I returned to running without
stopping.

I ran under a pedestrian overpass just before the finish and
heard such loud cheering for me and the other runners that I
felt like I was in the Olympics. It was intoxicating. I forgot
about all the pain I'd experienced. I summoned what little
energy I had left and sprinted to the finish line, where a
volunteer pulled a small, square tab with a round hole in it off
my race bib and threaded it over a string to record my time
and place in the race. I was exhausted and elated, but I
wanted to know where my friends were and how I would get
back to our hotel so I could lie down. After nearly an hour,
we found each other beyond the finish line and limped back
to the car together, detailing our races the whole way.

When we went to dinner that night, I could barely make it
down the stairs from the restaurant to the street. I had never
been so sore in my entire life. And the outrageous headache I
was battling did not go away until I barely managed to sip

down a single, watery beer with our meal. Yet I felt great. I was deeply proud of the accomplishment—one that was not even on my radar a few months prior.

Adding to my sense of triumph, I was accepted to the University of North Carolina School of Medicine that same month. I had done well enough on the MCATs that I decided to apply to a handful of medical schools scattered around the country. I reckoned that if I gained acceptance to one of them, I would go and fulfill my dream of becoming a doctor. If I faced rejection again as I had from CU in high school, I would have a PhD to finish as consolation.

Fortunately, my academic advisor was the chair of the Department of Epidemiology, where I was getting my public health degree. He had made the reverse switch years prior, going into epidemiology after just two years in medical school, realizing that taking care of patients was not for him. He was sympathetic to my desire to change and offered to award me a master's degree if I completed a publishable research project and one more semester of classes. So I took a job sitting at a computer, crunching numbers and writing code for statistical analysis software. It was an interesting challenge, but it was not for me. I wanted to interact with other people, not computers, to make a true difference in another person's life, to be on my feet and work with my hands. Looking back now, I realize that I likely would have been miserable at a desk job for an entire career. I shudder at the thought of staying in my program for five to seven years trying to get a PhD, only to come out on the other side with a job that didn't suit me.

My advisor kept his word when I came back to his office at the end of that summer break with a publishable paper. Just six weeks after finishing the marathon and getting into medical school, I successfully defended my thesis and earned a master's degree.

Enrolling in a master's degree program was a valuable way to bolster my medical school application and learn more about myself, about the things I liked and the things I didn't like. It also got me out of taking statistics in medical school—a small prize for eighteen months' worth of work.

After my public health degree was over, it was time to have fun for nine months until medical school started. I moved to Boulder for the first time, living with Vincent, Kevin, Luke, and Frank, a friend of Luke's from New Jersey. I went there to wait tables, ski, run, and party until medical school started. It was a fantastic time in my life. I had no responsibilities— no studying for classes, no writing a thesis, no applying to medical school, no entrance exams to take. It was the first and last time I would have such freedom. I enjoyed it to the fullest.

I met a fun group of women while working at the West End Tavern, a gritty bar known for great burgers, high-end tequila, cute waitresses, and an incredible rooftop view of Boulder's iconic Flatirons, a mesmerizing group of nearly parallel rock formations projecting toward the heavens and visible for scores of miles.

Steph was a standout among the attractive waitresses who worked at the West End. For years she had dated Jason, a friend of Kevin's, who sadly would succumb to the scourge of addiction later in life. She was known to be a free spirit and incredibly fun. We shared the same tastes in music and would see each other at concerts. Working, partying, and going to shows at Red Rocks with Steph and the others from the West End was easy. Living with the guys was a blast. We had constant fun partying, busting each other's balls, and heading up to the mountains to ski. Despite being friends with Luke and Vincent for ages, we had never lived together before, and it was only a matter of days before I knew why Luke was friends with Frank. He was riotous, sharp, and unassuming.

My first few months on the job at the West End, I found myself hungover nearly daily. As a food runner, I had to carry trays of food from the kitchen up to the rooftop and buckets of ice up two flights of stairs from the basement. It was a physically demanding job, but I loved being there, soaking up as well as contributing to the energy that kids in their early twenties exude. On occasion, when the weather was great and the rooftop was really cranking, our manager would stop the madness for a minute so we could all catch our breath. We would stand together in the tiny, enclosed portion of the bar on the roof and have a group toast, taking a shot of whiskey or tequila before going right back to work for the rest of the night. It was a far cry from writing code by myself in a computer lab.

That partying lifestyle ended abruptly the day I left the West End and drove back to North Carolina to start medical school. As much fun as working at the West End had been like many parts of my life, I knew it was a transitional period. The ultimate goal of becoming a physician and testing the absolute limits of my physical stamina and intellectual abilities lay ahead.

Chapter 3

Gunners

I returned to Chapel Hill in August 1997 and moved into an old yellow farmhouse on Franklin Street, a mile from campus with my sister Kristi, her husband, Andrew, and their daughter, Riley. We would live together for all four years I was in medical school. Andrew started law school in Chapel Hill the day I started medical school. We were lucky to be in school at the same time and have a close enough relationship to live together. I learned a lot about parenting from Kristi and Andrew, who were as patient as the day is long. Kristi was a great mom and kept the house together while I contributed little more than rent, jokes at dinner, and muscle to move the furniture every so often as Kristi changed her mind about the ideal location of the couch or TV. I tried to help out more when I could, but school kept me busy and they were very understanding about it.

One evening I babysat Riley while Kristi and Andrew went out to the movies for a much-needed break. Riley grew upset when her parents left and began to cry. I tried to calm her by feeding her a bottle, which she chugged down. But the crying resumed immediately afterward. I held Riley in my arms and bounced her up and down with deep knee bends, facing her away from me toward a standing mirror—a trick Kristi used on occasion to sooth her. Riley continued to cry, exhausting herself but not before projectile vomiting the milk she had just downed, leaving me scrambling to clean her, the mirror, and the floor. Finally, I put her to bed, and then being the exhausted medical student that I was, fell dead asleep.

Kristi was an anxious new mother at times and a caring sister, so she called to check in with me during the movie. When I didn't answer, Kristi went back into the theater and told Andrew, "We have to go. Something is wrong. Michael is not answering the phone. What if the house is on fire?"

They sped home, but when they got there, they found no flames. They did, however, find me facedown on top of my bed, fully clothed with the lights on. Riley was snug in her crib in a new set of pajamas. I felt terrible that they had to come home early. They paid for a real babysitter after that.

Medical school was an incredibly intense yet amazing experience. I met some of the best friends of my life there. Rod and Adair were a married couple who pulled off the rare feat of both gaining admission to the same medical school at the same time. Rod was from Colorado, so we had lots to talk about right away. He lived life larger than anyone I had ever met. He was inclined to spend every penny he had on having fun, every minute reaching for greatness. To sustain his manic pace, he drank more coffee in a day than I drank in a week. Adair was refined and poised, the product of a proper New England upbringing. She did not suffer fools gladly, although she put up with the antics that Rod and I got into most Friday nights after a long week of studying and exams. Adair started medical school walking with a cane, convalescing from a knee surgery, hoping she would run again one day. Being fit was as important to her as having fun was to Rod.

Parag was the jovial, confident, even-keeled son of doctors who immigrated from India and was the smartest kid in the room his whole life. He and I were in the same lab and spent endless hours shooting the shit and cracking jokes. I marveled at his confidence. Rod, Adair, and I were forced to study like maniacs to keep up with the demanding course load, while Parag would breeze through the material, leaving time to play golf, watch sports, or go see his mom, whom he referred to as his *best girl*. Parag had an unusual but entertaining habit of meandering around town with his shirt off, or "SO," as he called it after a few beers, even in the colder months. I loved him immediately.

Rod, Parag, and I became a trio of sorts, drinking together on the weekends, studying on occasion, and golfing when time and weather permitted. At the end of medical school, the three of us spent a month together in Chile with Vincent, backpacking through Torres del Paine National Park and adventuring in Pucón before heading our separate ways for residency. Having friends like Rod, Parag, and many others in medical school was a welcomed change from my lackluster social life after college.

Medical school was akin to a family road trip that never ended. The first two years in Chapel Hill, students were assigned to one of five labs. The labs were windowless rooms that housed desks where medical students kept their books and microscopes. While we spent about half our time in lectures with all two hundred students, the other half was spent with our assigned lab partners, doing anatomy dissections in the cadaver lab, reviewing pathology slides under high power, or studying in the lab between classes. The sheer number of hours spent together created a bond among us, whether we liked it or not.

The administration at the school of medicine was truly invested in the success of every student. If anyone needed help, they were there for them. They laid out everything in front of us and said, "Here is what you need to do to succeed." There were no mysteries. Anyone who didn't make the grade was a victim of the academic rigor, unfortunate circumstances, or their own negligence.

Even with this support, some couldn't take the pressure of medical school. One scholarship student announced in the first month that medical school would not be interfering with his social life. He failed out after one year. A whip-smart kid who could run a mile under four and a half minutes rarely showed up to class, opting to read the textbooks and syllabi instead. He quit a month into the third year in the middle of our OB/GYN rotation and became a schoolteacher. A few were smart but could not handle the volume. They were forced to decelerate, completing the first two academic years in three calendar years.

The diversity of our class was a far cry and a welcomed change from the very White worlds of CSU and Titusville, New Jersey. We had a large percentage of minority students. Slightly more than half the class was women, and lots of students were from North Carolina, ranging from the type of kids I knew at Ravenscroft to those who were the first in their families to attend college, much less medical school. In the labs, our assigned seats displayed a random assortment of sex, color, and privilege. In the lecture halls, though, I was struck by the distinct geographical divide in seating between my Black classmates and the rest. People typically sat in the same seats, which they had chosen at will and declared their spot for the duration of our first two years. Those seating choices, established early on, seemed to represent the diversity of not only races but also personality types. Many of our classmates of color chose to sit together early on, and it stuck for the remaining two years of lectures regardless of whatever friendships developed outside the lecture hall. The same held true for each student's academic attitude. The closer a student sat to the professors, the more likely that student was to brazenly declare themselves a candidate for achieving a grade of honors in each class. Rod and Adair sat in the front row next to one guy who kept his arms crossed at all times, never taking a single note for the entirety of our didactic years. He aced the exams. Parag and I sat next to each other like a married couple, a dozen rows back at the unofficial divide between the gunners and those students wanting to fly below the radar until the clinical years, or worse yet, those suffering from imposter syndrome who simply wanted to pass.

Our first final exam was just two weeks into our first semester. When we started medical school, I was three years removed from my undergraduate studies, where I had learned the basic sciences that form the foundation of medicine. In medical school, cell biology was brand new to me. Whereas my classmates seemed to know it already, I was either learning it for the first time or had forgotten everything I learned several years prior. Taking an exam for a final grade just fourteen days into medical school was nerve-racking. Grading was honors, pass, or fail. I was happy at that point to just get a *P* for pass. "P equals MD" was the refrain many of us uttered, just trying to get through the demanding course load.

Eventually, I would set my standards higher than just passing. In many ways, the competition was cutthroat. Only so many grades of honors were given out for each subject. That meant most students received a pass. Being a gunner meant being the type of student who went the extra mile, vying for honors at all costs. Closet gunners secretly studied far more than they let on, trying to convince the rest of us that they excelled without needing to study—a rare breed of super geniuses who might go on to be pediatric cardiothoracic surgeons or get a PhD while in medical school, launching their academic career.

For many of us, medical school was humbling. We were all used to being at the top of our college classes. That's how we got into medical school in the first place. Med school, however, gave you reason to question your intellectual superiority. There was always someone brighter than you sitting just a few seats away. To wit, I dated a woman who made it through college in just three years without ever getting lower than an A, and even she was not our class's top student. The combination of possessing superior intelligence and being a gunner put the select few at the top of the class. For most, that also meant success in the final two clinical years of medical school. For a few others, it did not translate

—the physical toll of the extreme hours got to them, or the translation of knowledge into practical implementation was a bridge too far. These students dropped out, failed out, or were asked to take time away or leave altogether because of their erratic behavior brought on by the stress and lack of sleep.

Despite the rigors of medical school, life outside the classroom went on for all of us. For me, it meant the illness of a dear friend. Partway through my first year of medical school, I got a call from Kevin about Ryan, whom we went to Europe with just a few years prior. Ryan woke up one day in Nederland with double vision. He went to see an eye doctor, which led to an MRI of his brain. There was a tumor. A biopsy showed it was cancerous. The location of the tumor made it inoperable. Ryan had just started dating someone who had every right in the world to make a beeline out of his life; this guy she barely knew was given a death sentence. Although she stuck it out for over a year, their relationship ended while Ryan was still battling the cancer.

Ryan had a positive attitude and was 100 percent convinced that he would pull through. But conviction wasn't enough to secure victory. We all gathered in Ryan's hospital room in Boulder when things got really bad. We cried and hugged each other while Ryan labored to breathe. He could still give us a thumbs-up at that point but couldn't communicate any more than that. My brief leave of absence from medical school to say goodbye to Ryan that week was the last time I saw him. He went home and hung on for a little while longer before dying in mid-May 1999.

His illness and our loss made me consider long and hard whether neurosurgery was a career option for me. On one hand, I could help people like my friend Ryan if and when a tumor could be removed. On the other, it was the opposite of being an obstetrician, where you are there for some of the most joyous moments of people's lives. It turns out neither would be my calling.

After several clinical rotations, I realized that orthopedic surgery seemed to fit me better than anything else. These decisions are made with precious little information, but I am certain I made the right choice. I never had any student rotations on specialties like dermatology, ophthalmology, or plastic surgery, which perhaps could have swayed my opinion. Likely that was for the best, although operating in the middle of the night sometimes makes me wish I had tried to be a dermatologist, where working nights and weekends is essentially unheard of.

I had great mentors in Chapel Hill, both in the administration and in orthopedic surgery. More than that, though, I had the full support of my classmate friends. Parag and our friend Aimee also decided to go into orthopedic surgery. Rod chose emergency medicine, and Adair became a psychiatrist. Our other friends ran the gamut of specialties. On Match Day, when we each found out where we would be spending the next several years training, almost all my friends got their first choices, myself included. We were each handed a box of wooden matches to represent Match Day as our futures were read aloud. My residency would be in Chicago at Northwestern University—a stunning departure from my languishing academic performance in high school.

That evening, we went out and celebrated getting through the hardest four years of our lives in anticipation of many more that would be even harder.

Chapter 4

Where Is Your Boyfriend?

Residency is perhaps the most challenging aspect of becoming a surgeon, and it's a grueling slog. While medical school is academically rigorous, being a resident adds to that with even longer work hours and the pressures of making quick life-or-death decisions. Thrust upon each resident is an amount of responsibility that constantly exceeds his or her level of knowledge and comfort. It is truly sink or swim. The system itself weeds out those not cut out for the demands the career puts on its partakers.

My internship, the first of my five years of residency, was packed with rotations on twelve different surgical specialties ranging from general surgery, where gallbladders and intestines are the main quarry, to plastic surgery, which included elective cosmetic procedures and complex reconstructive surgeries where muscles are moved from one part of the body to another to cover defects caused by trauma, cancer, or infection. Some rotations were directly applicable to being an orthopedic surgeon, while others simply taught us how to stay awake for two days straight or put up with massive egos.

Despite the intense schedule of my internship, I managed to run just enough during the first few months that I was able to race the Chicago Marathon during my neurosurgery rotation. Running allowed me to escape mentally from the rigors of work, and I used it to prove to myself that I could enjoy some part of my life outside the hospital. I was loath to admit that residency was the single most important thing in my life, although it was.

The week of the marathon, I was on call overnight and up from 4:00 a.m. Thursday until midnight on Friday. Although we would usually go home around 5:00 p.m. on Fridays, our senior resident, a certain breed of psychopath who prided himself on torturing younger residents, decided we should round as a team on the entire service of patients after we finished in the operating room that afternoon. Perhaps he had heard me say I would be racing that weekend. Or perhaps he was just sadistic. Regardless, I expected us to round briefly then be let free, but we kept going and going for hours without stopping.

"We are going to get to the bottom of every single detail on every goddam patient tonight," he barked.

This went beyond schadenfreude. This clearly was the result of him being derided by one of the attending neurosurgeons for something being missed on one of the patients. That something could have been life-threatening as easily as it could have been infinitesimally insignificant, but teaching attention to every single detail was the name of the game, especially for neurosurgery.

I could barely remain upright as we stood outside each patient's room discussing their care. I was so weary that the questions being hurled at me were unintelligible. Luckily, the senior resident's ire was shared among all the junior residents that night and not aimed solely at me as the intern. I made it home in the wee hours of Saturday morning and collapsed onto my futon in my four-hundred-square-foot studio apartment.

In those days, the world went completely black when I went to bed. I would fall asleep within seconds of my head hitting the pillow. There would be no dreams or nightmares aside from the ones I was living. My body did not toss or turn. I would wake up six to seven hours later in the same position I lay down in, still exhausted but ready to fight the day at hand. At times I felt like Don Quixote tilting at windmills I was so delirious. During the day I would fall asleep at any moment if I remained still for too long. This is the type of exhaustion that residency used to cause every budding surgeon. Times have changed since then, though, and those types of work hours have been outlawed—I think for the better. At some point we just got used to being that tired. It wasn't until the exhaustion went away that we realized it was even there.

Before graduating medical school, I began dating Jenn, a lovely, highly intelligent woman who lived in California. Adair introduced me to Jenn during our third year in Chapel Hill. She was a childhood friend of Adair's and had attended Yale and then the Medill School of Journalism at Northwestern years before my arrival in Chicago. Jenn flew in from California one week that first autumn of my residency to host clients at a chic restaurant in the River North neighborhood, halfway between the hospital and my humble studio apartment. She worked as an editor for one of the big three educational publishers. She was nice enough to bring me along to dinner, and I partook in the conversation by telling a couple of stories of my short time in medicine and listening to them discuss book publishing. I remained engaged and upright until the multiplicative effects of work and a single beer caused me to fall asleep while sitting at the table, my head bobbing in front of my body. Jenn's colleagues were nice enough to understand that I was a surgical intern working ungodly hours and kindly encouraged me to go get some sleep. Had I not been so dog-tired, I might have been embarrassed. Instead, I kissed Jenn goodbye, left the restaurant, and went straight home to my futon, where blackness fell upon me once again.

The sleep destitution continued for two years and affected everything in my life. I feel confident that I would have learned a lot more had I been awake and alert to see and hear what was going on at the hospital. At some point, that level of rigor affects everyone. Some dropped out. Some changed to kinder, gentler residency programs, like pediatrics or radiology. Others were asked to leave. I kept my head down throughout internship and made it to my second year — when our orthopedic training started in earnest — still alive.

At the start of our second year, my residency classmates and I met with our new chief resident, a guy a few years older than I was named Richard Bijou, and our department chairman, Dr. Thomas Muller, a gaunt man in his sixties and the longest-tenured chairman of orthopedics in the country. He had been at the helm for nearly thirty years and was the long-standing team doctor for a professional sports team. A childhood illness had weakened the muscles in both of his hands, which was clearly noticeable by shaking his hand, if not by the naked eye. It also seemingly affected his vocal cords given the constant strain in his voice. It was a marvel that he was able to operate at all given his lack of strength in his hands. Muller ran a tight ship, including making all the residents come to the hospital for an academic conference every Saturday, a punitive measure ensuring we all knew we were on a short leash from the word *go*. No absences were allowed from the conferences except during vacation. Period. This meant no weekends off for a four-year stretch.

Chief Resident Bijou was a short, nerdy-looking guy with thinning, tightly cropped hair who had been hand-selected by Muller to oversee the junior residents for the next six months, organizing conferences and keeping everyone in line. At our first meeting, the nine of us in our residency class were given an exam to test our proficiency and knowledge. It was a copy of the in-training exam given to all orthopedic residents at the end of each year of training. Muller prided himself on his residents doing particularly well on the exam, ranking consistently above the 90th percentile. When the test was handed to us, we were told to do our best. We had little experience with any of the material on the exam, so we were navigating uncharted waters.

Bijou left us alone in a room to take the test, and a murmur began to build. We had no chance of answering these questions accurately. What on earth was a Sauvé-Kapandji procedure? Who had ever heard of Kienbock's disease? At some point it was simply comical. We tried our best, but it was taking an eternity to answer each question.

After a couple of hours, Bijou returned.

"How is it going?" he asked.

"We have no idea what most of this stuff means," one guy answered honestly.

"How much more do you have left?" Bijou queried.

"We're barely halfway done," the guy said.

"Just hurry up. You don't have to put your names on it. This is just to see what you guys know."

Relieved, we finished and went on with what was left of our weekend. When we returned to work Monday, each of us had an assignment of a six-week rotation. Some were on the sports medicine service, some were at the children's hospital, one was on the spine service. Each morning, we would get to the hospital by 5:00 a.m., sometimes earlier, and round on the patients on our respective services. By 6:00 a.m., we would have to be at our daily meeting to cover one of a variety of orthopedic topics we would need to learn to treat patients — or more importantly for Muller, it seemed, to do well on the annual in-training exam. By 7:30 a.m., we would be in the operating room or starting to see patients in clinic.

At the end of the first week, Muller pulled all nine of us into a conference room to talk to us about the in-training sample test we had taken the Saturday before. I expected he would encourage us by saying he knew the test was over our heads but that he and Bijou, along with the rest of faculty, were there to teach us what we needed to know, the way we had been guided through medical school in Chapel Hill.

I was dead wrong.

"I have never been so disgusted with a class of residents in my entire career as I am right now," he said, his staccato, cracking voice filled with anger. "The fact that you guys didn't even put your names on these exams sickens me. You had better get your act together immediately, or I will throw your asses out of this program."

I was bemused. Bijou was standing right there beside him. Why wasn't he saying that he told us not to put our names on the exams? That we gave a solid effort?

Muller left and Bijou, the traitor, barked, "I don't want to hear another fucking word about this," his face filled with contempt. Then he walked out, slamming the door behind him.

We stared at each other, bewildered by our feckless chief resident's inaction. These were the men who would oversee our education and control whether we passed on to the next year of training. What had I gotten myself into? Why on earth did I choose this residency program? I lost all respect for Bijou that day. I would have to make it through my training that year in spite of Bijou, not because of him. Thankfully, we had a lot of talented surgeons at Northwestern to learn from who would make up for our lack of leadership.

The decisions that go into choosing a medical specialty or the place where training for said specialty is done are made with a limited knowledge of the reality that lies ahead. My decision to rank Northwestern as my first choice is a prime example, being based on a single visit to the program. Sometimes the decisions of what and where are made for you. Your plastic surgeon may have wanted to be an ophthalmologist but wasn't accepted to such a program. Or she may have wanted to train at UCLA in sunny Southern California but was accepted at her fifth or sixth choice, somewhere in the Pacific Northwest. Further, she may have enjoyed a career in dermatology most but was never exposed to it in medical school — or even made her decision to become a plastic surgeon based on a TV show. Such vagaries went into most of our choices when it came to both specialty selection and residency.

For me, it started in medical school when I spent a month at the University of New Mexico and a month at the University of Utah on the orthopedics services. New Mexico was chaotically overwhelming with the amount and severity of trauma. Albuquerque sits at the crossroads of I-25 and I-40 in an area with plenty of alcohol, drug, and gang activity. We saw people thrown from moving vehicles, others who had been hit in the head with hammers, and an endless number of drunk driving accidents. The University of Utah, in comparison, was a great mix of trauma and elective surgery. In both places, I found surgeries that I enjoyed being a part of, patients I liked caring for, and residents whose personalities meshed well with mine.

I interviewed at several other programs, including Harvard, where I got the sense that the residents worked more hours than any other place in the nation. I believed they came out well trained but probably divorced if they were married going in. When I interviewed with Northwestern, I was impressed with the program. The residents seemed happy and smart. The hospital was a brand-new state-of-the-art facility. It was gorgeous. At the time, it was the most expensive building ever constructed in Chicago and one of the largest orthopedic residencies in the nation in a large city. I ranked it first, wanting to have an urban experience for once in my life and thinking that if I had to work a hundred hours per week, it would be nice to do so in an impeccable hospital.

I found a new set of friends in residency, reinforcing my suspicion that some situations are better than others for making close relationships. Joe was an Ivy Leaguer of Indian descent who was fun to hang out with, similar in many ways to Parag. Cary was a smart, hilarious Midwesterner who reminded me of Rod. Flores was a savant who could remember just about anything he had ever read, but I couldn't say I had an old friend he reminded me of. My other residency classmates were a mix of nerdy, cocky, and eccentric characters, not dissimilar to those in medical school, but each of these guys (there were no women my year) had finished at the top of their classes in order to get into orthopedics.

Ultimately, I got a lot out of my residency, including a vast knowledge of orthopedics, a tolerance to working an ungodly number of hours, and the surgical skills needed to operate proficiently and build upon once in practice.

I also happened upon the love of my life.

Three months into my internship on my fourth rotation, transplant surgery, I met Melissa Cellucci. I was on service with another intern, Amanda, whom I had been with on the cardiothoracic surgery rotation two months prior. Amanda had already proved herself to be far more competent and confident than I felt I was. A former Dallas Cowboys cheerleader who was in the urology residency—truly a man's world—she was ready to prove everyone wrong. She insisted that everyone address her as Dr. Bellerose in the hospital, which was not the norm for the interns and put me on the defensive at times.

Amanda and I met Melissa early in the rotation. She was one of several inpatient solid organ transplant coordinators. As a transplant nurse, she was tasked with managing the daily inpatient care of the kidney, liver, and pancreas transplant patients and the kidney and liver donors. She ordered and reviewed their labs, ensured they were on the correct medications and dosages, ordered and followed up on necessary tests, collaborated with the other specialists, and executed discharge planning. She lightened the loads of her fellows and attendings—which she did with her smile as much as with her wit.

As interns, we rounded on the patients with the transplant coordinators, seeing them each morning bright and early, then presented our findings to the transplant fellows or the attending surgeons. We answered constant pages from the floor nurses, day and night. We tried to help the transplant coordinators, but in many instances, they knew more than we did and were teaching us.

It was hard to outshine Amanda, given her dedication and smarts. Most days I did not dare try to show her up—except when it came to Melissa. The day we met I was in the transplant conference room looking at the images of a patient's CT scan. Melissa walked in the room and our eyes met. *Wow*, I thought. *She is gorgeous*. She had cocoa brown hair cut above her shoulders, dark brown eyes, eyebrows to match, and the cutest little smile that rose slightly higher on the left side.

She introduced herself with confidence. "Hi. I'm Melissa. Who are *you*?" I could tell right away she was smart, fiery, and ambitious. Melissa had been living in Chicago and working at Northwestern for nine months. After finishing her nursing degree at the University of Virginia, she worked as a general medicine nurse at Johns Hopkins. She later became a transplant coordinator at the University of Maryland, a high-volume center with great demands on the nurse coordinators.

Melissa shined in the transplant program there and used it as a springboard to come to Northwestern's transplant program. She was living with her best friend from college, Julie, and was dating a urology resident a couple of years older than she was.

While I happened to be in a long-distance relationship with Jenn and thought the world of her, I didn't feel the kind of spark with her that made me believe we should stay together forever.

I did feel a spark with Melissa, though. It was easy and fun to talk and work with her. I told Vincent that I had met a woman I desperately wanted to date but that she was dating someone else. I considered all the options and took a flyer on asking her out for a drink after work.

Melissa said, "Sure! I will bring my boyfriend."

It sounded like it would be very awkward. But I couldn't back out at that point. I picked a bar close to my apartment, and we agreed to meet at 8:00 p.m. Melissa beat me there, which I would later come to learn was an anomaly for her. I came in and sat next to her at the bar. She looked beautiful. That hair. Those eyes.

"Where is your boyfriend?" I asked.

"He's not coming. He said he was tired."

Perfect.

We enjoyed each other's company sitting and talking and drinking our beers. We decided to meet again a week or two later, this time at a bar a block from work that regularly served the Northwestern Hospital staff. We sat in a corner at a small table in the darkest part of the bar. We laughed and talked and flirted. Eventually, Melissa went to the bathroom, and when she came back, she had a shirt in her hand, which she did not have when she left the table or entered the bathroom. It was a faded, light purple shirt with a yellow oval surrounding a red star.

"What is that?" I asked.

"A T-shirt. I found it on the floor next to the toilet," she said.

"What? You found a shirt next to the toilet and you took it?"

"Yeah. Isn't it awesome?"

"Gross!" I said, laughing. I figured she might be eccentric or perhaps a hoarder, but I put it out of my mind.

The next morning, I awoke early as always and met Amanda to see all the patients. We made our way through each of them, preparing to present to the attending surgeons on rounds. Melissa presumably slept in as she was working a shift that started at 8:00 a.m. She joined us in the middle of our rounds as we were presenting one of the patients who had received kidney and pancreas transplantations three nights prior. She listened intently, detailing the patient's lab values from the yellow flow sheets when asked.

Melissa and I made eye contact with each other for a few fleeting moments. Once it was my turn to present the next patient to the rest of the transplant team, Melissa smiled at me as she unbuttoned her white lab coat, revealing the T-shirt with the oval and star that she found the night before. I quickly turned away, trying my best to not laugh and to remain focused and discuss the current status of the patient whose room we were standing outside of. My attraction to her doubled in that moment. Hoarder or not, it would be worth being with her.

We began to see each other more frequently. One night, Melissa was out with friends and was planning to come to my apartment afterward. I waited for her past the time she said she was coming. Eventually she showed up, flustered.

"I got pulled over on the way here," she said.

"Oh, no. What happened?"

"I accidentally ran through a stop sign. I was anxious to get here," she said. The words were titillating to me. "And I was in the middle of taking a hit of pot."

"Oh, boy."

"I kept driving until I could blow the smoke out the passenger window where the cop wouldn't see the plume.

Then when the cop pulled me over, I didn't have my license with me. I'd also let my insurance expire. He was a total jerk at the station. He made me wait and wait and wait. Finally, I stood up and asked what was taking so long. He yelled at me to sit down, but a few minutes later, he let me go. I just need to get my proof of registration, and they will drop the ticket for that."

Perhaps the T-shirt had been a sign. I started wondering whether Melissa was unhinged. How was she so organized and professional at work? I considered ending our relationship before it even began. But Melissa's beauty and spirit were irresistible. I told her how I felt about her, and she told me she felt the same way about me. After our conversation, she ended her relationship with her boyfriend. I ended mine with Jenn at the same time.

We began to date, but kept it quiet at work for months at Melissa's request. The hospital could be a small world despite its massive size.

We went to the *Van Gogh and Gauguin: The Studio of the South* exhibit at the Art Institute of Chicago on our first official date. It was breathtaking. So was she. I reached out for Melissa's hand as we navigated through the crowds from painting to painting. We both knew this exhibit and our relationship were something very special.

As the weeks passed, I moved on to other rotations, keeping my head down to get through internship and on to the orthopedic part of my residency. A year and a half after our first date, Melissa and I took a trip to see Vincent in Argentina. The trip had been planned for Vincent's wedding. Before we got there, though, Vincent said there would be no nuptials. With plane tickets already in hand, we used it as a vacation to go visit my friend in his new home. When we got there, we discovered that Vincent and his fiancée, Lorena, were still together despite the canceled wedding.

Things seemed copacetic between Vincent and Lorena when we arrived. Melissa and I had dinner out with them and stayed in a hotel the first night. The exchange rate put the three-course steak and fish dinner with wine for four of us at around thirty dollars. On a resident's salary, it was liberating to eat and drink for so little.

The second day, the four of us drove for several hours in Vincent's Defender through the pampas outside town toward a lake abutting massive sand dunes in front of small, arid mountains. Once at the lake, Vincent dropped Melissa and me off at a house he'd rented for us at the water's edge. It was ideal. Not fully understanding the situation Vincent was in with Lorena, I had planned to use our trip to Argentina to propose to Melissa.

That day, Melissa and I went canoeing into one of the lake's secluded coves. As I began to get down on one knee to propose, our canoe lost its makeshift mooring on the rocks we were on and began to float away. Distracted by the canoe, I stood up and chased after it, giving Melissa a moment to consider what might be about to happen and ruining the surprise. I returned to Melissa atop the rocks and got on one knee in earnest, me in my board shorts, Melissa in her cute little bikini, and finished the proposal. Melissa teared up and said yes, and we savored each moment of the trip on the water back to the dock.

When we saw Vincent and Lorena that afternoon, we announced that we were engaged. Vincent seemed genuinely happy for us. Lorena, however, did not. Later that evening, Lorena left the lake and drove Vincent's Defender the three hours back to San Rafael. Without us. Vincent, ever even-keeled and capable, explained the situation to us without worry, then secured us a ride home with a local the next day. But he asked us not to bring up the engagement in front of Lorena again. Melissa and I were unsure what to make of the entire situation.

Lorena and Vincent eventually married, and Lorena became pregnant with their only child. Vincent planned on bringing Lorena to the United States for their child to be born, giving him instant US citizenship. Those plans were ruined in an unimaginable way. Just a month before Lorena gave birth, her father killed her mother and then himself.

Vincent hired two local men to clean up Lorena's parents' house after the bodies were removed. This involved the gruesome task of cleaning the spray of blood, teeth, and hair from the walls and ceilings from the shotgun blasts. Vincent dealt with the trauma as best he could, but the marriage ended just a year after his son was born. Committed to fatherhood, Vincent stayed in Argentina.

As for Melissa and me, we remained in separate apartments, enjoying a romantic engagement through the spring and summer in Chicago. Our busy schedules still allowed us to spend time together as we planned our wedding and dreamed of our new lives together.

We wed nine months after our engagement on a stunningly beautiful day in Massachusetts in September 2003. Like our engagement in Argentina and many other parts of my life, our wedding day was punctuated by drama.

Chapter 5

The Best Man

A year into my residency, just after my intern year, I brought Melissa to meet Kevin for our thirtieth birthday. She had heard a lot about Kevin from me and had spoken with him on the phone a few times. We flew to Denver, where Kevin and his wife, Meghan, picked us up. The car ride back to the house from the airport seemed a little odd with long periods of silence, but I didn't think too much of it. When we got to their house, however, their behavior confirmed my suspicions that something was amiss. I heard Kevin coughing a lot upstairs, and I smelled something sweet burning. Kevin played it off as though he'd lit a match in the bathroom to get the smell out. I didn't buy it.

"Kevin is on drugs," I told Melissa during one of his trips upstairs to the second floor that first day.

"What?" she asked. "What do you mean?"

"I can just tell. Something is not right."

"Yeah, the car ride seemed a little weird, but I never met your brother before."

Minutes later, Vincent arrived at the house. As we sat around talking, Kevin and Meghan nervously entered and exited the family room. I took Vincent aside and probed him for answers.

"I've been meaning to say something to you," he said sheepishly. "Kevin and Meghan are in deep on heroin."

"Heroin!" I exclaimed.

"Yeah. I should have called you up and said something to you earlier."

Vincent had been back in Boulder for a few months kayaking and occasionally partying with Kevin and Meghan. He explained that a few people in their social circle had started using heroin and that Kevin and Meghan had become addicted.

"Fuck." I paused. "Okay. We have to have an intervention," I said, not knowing what the hell I was even talking about.

The plan for the weekend had been to go up to Meghan's parents' condo in the mountains with her sister and Vincent. Melissa, Vincent, and I drove up there together. That evening, I spoke with Meghan's sister about the situation. She was totally unaware of what was going on, despite living in Denver and seeing the couple frequently. She was younger and a lot more innocent. While the religious aspect of her life was not what it once was, the puritan lifestyle was. This was totally foreign to her. I told her I would handle speaking with the couple.

What transpired that night was utterly uncomfortable. I confronted Kevin and Meghan in front of everyone.

"It is obvious that you guys are addicted to drugs," I said. I was not subtle, nor was I beating around the bush. I was beating them over the head with the truth. I would later learn how awful this approach is for someone not ready to hear the message you are giving them, be it patient or addict.

"We know how bad it's gotten," Vincent added.

Kevin's eyes locked in on mine for a millisecond, then darted to the floor. "You don't know what you're talking about."

Meghan sat silently and said nothing as she stared empty-eyed at the wall.

They denied the drug use. They made excuses. They lied. Then they locked themselves in the bedroom and did not come out for twenty-four hours, whereupon they drove straight back to Denver to find their dealer. They were each facing the horrible prospect of physical withdrawal, which they had been through before with each attempt to stop using. They were indeed in deep.

The couple had both been working at high-paying corporate jobs for several years, building wealth and status. But I found out that Kevin was not on vacation as he had told me; he'd been fired. His work suspected drug use because of his turbulent behavior and took away his badge access to the office. Meghan was clinging to a job by working odd hours, still getting most of her work done, albeit when no one was around to see how bad she looked.

I urged Kevin to go to rehab.

"This is really serious, Kevin. You are in over your head."

"It's fine. Vincent is exaggerating." It was one of his many excuses to keep using.

"It's not fine! You could die from this."

We kept the pressure on him from afar with phone calls from Chicago, and he relented after several weeks. He landed at an expensive rehab in Arizona, using $30,000 of his savings on the four-week stay. The final week was intended for family members to attend. People who deal with addiction need a ton of support from family and friends, particularly because many have emotional problems that stem from childhood. As a result, this addiction center got the family involved to confront certain matters, to try to resolve problems, and to offer advice on supporting someone who is trying to achieve or maintain sobriety.

Kevin called and pleaded with me to tell his counselors that we would not attend the family week. My parents were not particularly interested in it anyway, and I was unable to leave work. So Kevin left rehab a week early. I bought his convincing argument that he was sober and breathed a sigh of relief. *Thank God he did not overdose and die before we intervened,* I thought. I was naïve.

It soon became apparent that Kevin was using again. It turns out it took only a few hours. I had no experience dealing with an addict, so I fully expected him to stay sober after one crack at it. Within months he returned to another expensive rehab, draining more of his savings. He was spending tons of money on drugs alone. Another relapse after his second stint in rehab motivated me to start looking for extra assistance. I was feeling helpless and called a college roommate of ours to drive down to Denver from Fort Collins to intervene. Kevin convinced our friend to use drugs with him, though, foiling my plan to get him help. He was a tornado, sucking up and destroying everything in his path.

Inside of a year, their savings account was nearly empty. Their marriage began to splinter. Eventually they were forced to sell their house. They maxed out their credit cards and liquidated some of their retirement plans. Several hundred thousand dollars went to waste on their drug use and stints in posh rehabs.

When Melissa and I got engaged, I asked Kevin to be my best man. It was a risk; I knew he might show up in rough shape. I spoke with him several times in the weeks leading up to the wedding, and he assured me he would not be a liability. Just days before the wedding, he called.

"I am not going to make it to the wedding," he said.

I expected these words to come, though I had held out hope they would not.

"I understand. I just want you alive and healthy. I am so worried you're going to overdose."

"Don't worry, dude. I am fine."

I knew this was just another lie that I was going to have to live with. Our parents sent our friends and relatives an email telling them Kevin would not be at the wedding and asking them not to discuss his absence there. I believe they did it to allow Melissa and me to enjoy our wedding day as much as they did it to avoid answering painful questions. I felt worse for my parents than I did for me by far.

Kevin's impending truancy presented me with a difficult decision. I had to choose a new best man posthaste. My mother encouraged me to ask my father. In recent years, since my dad's retirement, he had mellowed and become very supportive of my career and me. But our relationship was still not necessarily up to best man standards. I considered each of my friends and felt choosing one over another was even more difficult. Ultimately, I asked my father. He was honored.

Our wedding was an amazing day with picture-perfect weather and scenery. Melissa's parents went all out, paying for the best of everything. The food and music were spectacular. Friends and family from far and wide came to celebrate the special day with us. I felt some pain about Kevin not being there as my best man, but more than anything, I just wanted him alive.

Over the next year and a half, Kevin went to a fourth, then fifth, then sixth rehab with the last vestiges of his retirement savings, credit cards, and help from our sister Kelly. One facility put him under general anesthesia for a rapid detoxification to avoid the horrible withdrawal symptoms that plague heroin users. Another rehab was in Antigua, founded by Eric Clapton. The seventh and final rehab was in California. Kevin, continuing his destructive path, used drugs inside that rehab facility with a counselor and other patients. He convinced another patient to loan him his car to get more drugs. The car broke down on his way, and Kevin simply abandoned it on the side of the road. He was unstoppable.

Our sister, Kelly, was living in San Francisco at that time with her husband, Tiff, and son, Charles. Kevin made his way down to the Bay Area and for the next year or so showed up periodically at Kelly and Tiff's house, asking for support. He lived in an apartment at first, then moved into a shipping container across the bay in Oakland with a bunch of Burner tweakers who spent days on end awake, building massive, steampunk sculptures for Burning Man. Once he ran out of money, he could no longer pay the tolls to cross the Bay Bridge or his parking tickets. His truck got impounded.

Taking Kelly and Tiff's advice, he decided to attend AA, where he met a girl. Before long, she went from a recovering alcoholic to heroin addict with Kevin. He became an Uber driver of sorts for his illegal alien heroin dealer in exchange for drugs. His dealer asked him to marry his sister as a path to citizenship. Kevin even swallowed bags of heroin to avoid arrest on one occasion.

Throughout this ordeal, I spoke to Kevin less and less. He would go months without calling me, and I had no way to call him. Kelly would update me if she saw Kevin, telling me how bad he looked or how desperately he begged for money. It got to the point that every time my phone rang, I feared someone was calling me to tell me that Kevin was dead. Kelly tried repeatedly to help him, but he was not prepared to change. As shocking as it seemed, he had not hit rock bottom.

Eventually, Kelly refused to be taken advantage of anymore. Trying to deal with Kevin's behavior while managing her own family's safety was causing her a lot of anxiety. So

Kevin got on a plane to Chicago. Melissa had pleaded with me to have Kevin come live with us, fearing that if he died, it would crush my spirit. Kevin told me he used frequent flyer miles, but I wasn't sure I could believe him. Like many other addicts, he had become a brazen liar and extremely manipulative. On occasion he would call me with some scam he was trying to pull off, begging me to get him a fancy hotel room in San Francisco to con someone into fronting him drugs without payment. I never felt like I could trust him.

When he showed up at our house, he held a clean, new suitcase, which could not possibly have been his, although his filthy, raggedy clothes were inside it. He was the skinniest I had ever seen him. He was unkempt. His clothes hung baggily off him. He smelled of cigarettes. His skin looked ashen. He had scabs all over his arms. Worse, he was completely out of it. Having a normal conversation with him was nearly impossible. He shifted around, never making eye contact or holding still. He immediately asked us for money. Melissa and I said no. "If you want something," I told him, "we will get it for you. Instead of giving you five bucks for a pack of cigarettes, we will go buy it for you. We can't trust you with money."

"But I need money to go to AA meetings. They expect you to give a donation," he retorted.

"You can have a dollar each time you go to a meeting," I said. We felt guilty about not trusting him with as little as $5, but knew better.

He had no bargaining power, so the arrangement stuck. At our behest, he saw an addiction specialist who put him on suboxone, a medication used to temper withdrawal symptoms from opioids. He started going to AA meetings every day. He stayed in our guest bedroom just off the kitchen, spending most of his time desperately trying to sleep the first few weeks. His eating habits were as bizarre as his behavior. We bought him pint after pint of Ben & Jerry's Cherry Garcia and Chunky Monkey ice cream. We found drips of it from the kitchen across the floor into his bedroom. Mustard was smeared all over the counter when he made a sandwich. We had to clean the toilet daily, which was beyond disgusting from the unavoidable diarrhea that opiate withdrawal causes.

We were just a year into our marriage when Melissa suggested we take Kevin in. We were both working long hours. We were both very driven, neat, ambitious people and pedantic about the house rules. Kevin thought we were as nuts as we thought he was. But he was a shell of his former self. He would be asleep when we left for work. He would be sitting on the couch staring off into space or on the back porch smoking a cigarette when we got home.

"I'll never know the brother I grew up with," I bemoaned nearly six months into his stay with us.

"What are we going to do with him?" Melissa asked me.

"As long as he can stay sober, we'll figure something out."

"That's not enough. He has to get a job," Melissa said firmly.

"I doubt he can work. Look at him."

"He can't just sit on the couch forever. He needs some responsibility. It will be good for him."

I doubted Melissa's tactic, but she was right. I was being too soft on Kevin. We made our demands clear: He had to start looking for a job and continue to go to AA meetings. Kevin's first step was to get his résumé together. He'd had a successful career until he was fired, but now there was a couple-year gap to account for. He would have to explain that part as an entrepreneurial experience of some sort. Perhaps flipping houses, which he had done, in essence with the house he'd owned. He cut his hair, shaved, gained back a lot of the weight he had lost, and put on a suit. United Airlines, based in Chicago, was hiring after they had just declared bankruptcy and were not the most sought-after place to work. He found a position as an economist. I was shocked he found gainful employment so quickly.

Kevin toughed it out for several years with United, dealing with a boss who made him constantly consider quitting. He kept up with his AA meetings in Chicago and then found another job in Colorado. He continued having great success in his career, stayed sober, and became even better than his old self. Eventually, we became best friends again.

DRUG AND ALCOHOL ADDICTION DIDN'T END IN OUR family with Kevin. Several years later, while visiting Kristi, Melissa and I noticed the telltale signs of drug use. My normally vivacious, athletic sister was gaunt and seemed anesthetized. Her pupils were microdots. Her gaze was fixed. Throughout high school and college, Kristi had been a little Goody Two-shoes, never even trying a cigarette and rarely, if ever, drinking. She likely never tried a single illicit drug.

After having kids, though, she developed abdominal pain and headaches. One doctor suggested she might be depressed. Another suspected she had irritable bowel syndrome. Her obstetrician recommended she take Fioricet, a medicine that contains a barbiturate, to control her pain. Her husband, Andrew, wasn't sure what to make of her declining health, but never suspected drug abuse. Kristi had been the picture of ideal health for years, running marathons and eating well. She was also a social butterfly with a tight-knit group of friends, most of whom had children of similar ages to hers.

Several months after our visit, Kristi admitted to Andrew she had become addicted to the pain meds. They suppressed her appetite and numbed her mind. Her girls were still young and just thought their mom needed to sleep a lot. Despite all these issues, Andrew's immediate reaction was one of relief that this wasn't something incurable like brain cancer. With the help of counselors, Kristi was able to get off the Fioricet but soon supplanted that with alcohol. This increased after the death of our father in 2012.

The next several years were tumultuous and ended in her asking for a divorce. Her troubles only worsened from there. Andrew soon had full custody of the girls, and Kristi was volleying back and forth between sobriety and drunkenness. She bounced from job to job and dreamt up one career idea after another, perhaps trying to figure out her new identity. She had gone from dedicated supermom to divorced part-time parent who needed to support herself after a long break from a once-flourishing career.

Kristi's four daughters grew up dealing with the pain of having an alcoholic mother. At times they played caretaker for her. Other times, for their own mental well-being, they stayed away without speaking to her for months. Like Kevin during his years using drugs and alcohol, Kristi habitually lied and manipulated others to get what she wanted. Along with alcoholism and drug abuse, she developed a growing spending addiction. Like Kevin, she went broke, only she did so at age fifty, when career prospects become dim.

She took advantage of our mother's generosity and spoiled her relationships with her siblings. The sister I lived with for four years during medical school became a stranger. When she realized she had squandered so much in her life, she began to drink recklessly. Just the same way I had with Kevin fifteen years prior, every time the phone would ring, I expected it to be someone calling to tell me Kristi was dead.

Addiction is a disease. I believe Kevin's addiction stemmed partly from pain he was dealing with and partly from bad choices. He had been hanging around a group of people who lived a party lifestyle, going to see music and doing drugs like cocaine before, during, and after the concerts to keep the party going all night. A few tried heroin, and that was it. Some struggled, but managed to kick the habit quickly. Kevin and his wife got in over their heads.

With Kristi, I never fully understood the demons she battled. My family certainly may have some genetic predisposition to addiction. Growing up under my father's roof may have taken an unfortunate psychological toll on us, as well. I think it's more complicated than that, though. Life is full of stresses that everyone handles differently. Bad shit happens to some people that doesn't happen to others. I have not battled addiction to drugs or alcohol, yet my twin brother can never have another drink again.

I have an uncanny number of friends who have had issues with addiction, whether they have dealt with them or not. I have seen abuse and addiction do everything from keeping people from achieving what they were truly capable of to destroying lives. Trying heroin is a choice. You can't get addicted if you don't try it. It sounds simple, but it's not so straightforward for everyone. Those who battle addiction are dealing with more than simply drinking or using. I have been to AA meetings with Kevin and have heard many heartbreaking stories. I've also been to Al-Anon meetings and witnessed the toll addiction has taken on the families of addicts. I would later recognize striking similarities between what alcoholism and ME can do to families. Job losses. Destitution. Divorce. Failing health. Abandonment. I wouldn't wish either condition on anyone.

Chapter 6

You Fucking Doctors

Kevin moved out after a year of living with us and got his own apartment in Bucktown, a trendy neighborhood of Chicago where Melissa had lived when I met her. He officially divorced Meghan after years of being estranged. Then he broke one of the unwritten rules of AA and started dating during his first year of sobriety. Grace was nine years younger than he was and seemed very put together. At first, I couldn't understand what she saw in the mess that Kevin was, but their relationship blossomed.

Melissa and I stayed in our apartment after Kevin moved out, enjoying what Chicago had to offer. Melissa was promoted to the lead transplant coordinator and began working even longer hours. I was so proud of her. The transplant surgeons loved her. Orthopedics stopped sending their residents to transplant surgery during internship, so I had made it to transplant and met Melissa just in time.

Residency became more tolerable as the years went by. Each fall I squeezed in enough time to run a marathon on just enough training to finish without having to walk as I had in my first marathon. My final year of residency, I signed up for Ironman Wisconsin, a 140.6-mile triathlon that involves a 2.4-mile swim and then a 112-mile bike ride, followed by a marathon.

I had seen the Hawai'i Ironman on TV in medical school, and it captured my imagination. My fourth year of residency, I drove up to Wisconsin to witness the Ironman as a spectator and decided on the spot to sign up for the following year. When I got back, I bought a triathlon bike and began my training. Most people would probably start with a shorter race, but as I had done with other things in life, I said, "Fuck it," and went all in.

To train for swimming, I used the YMCA pool and went from barely being able to swim one lap to becoming an efficient swimmer capable of the 2.4 miles with the help of a DVD on swim techniques. Once the weather warmed, I practiced open-water swimming with a wetsuit at Ohio Street Beach in Lake Michigan, just down the street from the hospital where I worked, adjusting to the seasickness that came from being in the lake and dealing with the small swells.

Because I lived in the heart of the city, I drove to the suburbs of Chicago to bike, where I discovered a beautiful countryside filled with horse farms in towns I never knew existed, like Barrington Hills and Algonquin. I also spent time on the actual racecourse outside Madison, a forty-mile loop of hilly pastoral farmland, beginning and ending in the town of Verona.

During many of my training rides, I developed a cough that became increasingly disabling. At first, I thought it was from asthma or perhaps a lack of biking fitness. It never seemed to happen until three or four hours into a ride. I noticed it happened more after I ate but that it also coincided with me getting close to exhaustion. I saw a doctor who treated me for both reflux and asthma.

The cough was excruciating at times, and some days I pedaled at an achingly slow pace for ten to twenty miles to get back to the car, sputtering the whole way. No matter the cause, I could not completely get rid of the symptoms and ended up on inhaled steroids, albuterol, and a proton pump inhibitor. It seemed like a lot just to be able to do a triathlon. I never suffered from any of this in my marathons and wondered why biking was so different.

Before the Ironman, I did my first Half Ironman—the Dairyland Triathlon in Racine, Wisconsin—in nearly 100-degree weather. I swam fairly well that day, but as I got out of the water, my left calf cramped to the point that I yelped and started limping. A spectator yelled at me, "Just keep going!" I heeded her warning and got on the bike. I began pedaling and soon found myself being passed by a constant stream of athletes of all shapes, sizes, and ages for the next three hours. I had no idea I was that bad of a cyclist. I checked to make sure my brakes were not rubbing and slowing me down, but it was me that was the problem. This was a total, unwelcomed revelation.

I managed to finish the bike and got to the run, ready to rock and roll. My calf cramp was long gone, and I started picking off the runners in front of me one by one. Running was clearly my strong suit. Despite the inferno, I kept moving. At mile seven, I began to overheat. The aid stations were equipped with cups of ice water that I dumped over my head. No drink, drug, or moment of passion had ever brought more ecstasy. It was the time between the aid stations, though, that shook my confidence. I finished the race and realized that going *twice* that length was beyond my ability. Not one to back down from a challenge, or perhaps driven by a fear of failure, I pressed on and kept training.

I made it to the start line in Madison on what would turn out to be a day that was just a few degrees cooler than my Half Ironman, but with 25 mph winds. It was like running in front of a hairdryer. The swim in Lake Monona started promptly at 7:00 a.m. From then, triathletes had until midnight to make it to the finish line. I was concerned only about biking fast enough to make the cutoff without my cough affecting my performance.

As soon as the cannon sounded to start the race, I realized I was in grave trouble. I was immediately pummeled by the arms and legs of the swimmers around me. In total, there were two thousand swimmers—and it felt like all eight thousand hands and feet were throwing haymakers and scissor kicks directly at my head. I could barely stay afloat. I began to get out of breath. My goggles got knocked cockeyed, filling one side with dark, murky water.

I thought I was going to drown.

I changed tack as quickly as possible and swam hard to the right to extricate myself from the melee. I floated on my back like a wounded otter for a few minutes and caught my breath, thinking, *This goddam race is over, and I'm only five minutes into it!*

I regained my composure, turned facedown into the black water, and began making strokes. I got into a rhythm, completed the two compulsory laps, and got out of the water after more than an hour. Because our wetsuits were difficult to take off, volunteers known as wetsuit strippers would violently pull them off as the triathletes sat on the ground, trying not to be dragged with the neoprene across the steamy pavement. We then had to retrieve our bikes on the upper parking level of the nearby convention center, Monona Terrace.

Unlike the start of the swim, the bike portion of the race began well. Because I'd trained several times on the gorgeous, rural course, I was able to keep up with many of the other cyclists. By one hundred miles in, however, I began to wither. I was dehydrated, undernourished, and overheated. I got off my bike, sat on the curb, and ate a Clif Bar, debating my fate. *What the hell am I doing here?* I wondered.

With no other way to get back to Melissa and my car, I was forced to ride my bike back to town and admit defeat. I struggled mightily riding the last hundred yards up the helix to the top of Monona Terrace, where a volunteer took my bike from me, and I went inside to call it quits. Unlike other triathlons, Ironman Wisconsin had an indoor transition area instead of a field or a series of tents. The air-conditioned convention center felt nearly as amazing as the ice water on my head had weeks before in Racine. I sat down, feeling trounced and contemplating what exactly went wrong. Next to me, a graying, sinewy man was squawking in a country accent, "My feet are burnin'!" I wanted to make him aware that the duct tape adhered to the skin of his heels undoubtedly was adding to that unpleasant sensation, but I was too tired to say anything.

After fifteen minutes, the man with the taped-up feet got up and headed out for the run. I simply could not let that wounded-looking man keep going while I quit. So I slipped on my running shoes, slowly got up from the plastic folding chair that supported my wilted body, and followed him out into the hot afternoon sun.

Even with Melissa there to cheer me on, I barely plodded along, exhausted in the nearly unbearable heat and wind. Soon, the familiar, awful discomfort in my chest began to surface. I pulled out my inhaler and took a deep breath, holding it to get the full load of medicine into my lungs. I became immediately, fantastically dizzy. The world started disappearing. *The inhaler is killing me!* I thought. I sat down. Then lay down. The earth seemed to be spinning off its axis to my weary brain. I had nearly twenty miles to go. Twenty. Damn. Miles.

I sat back up when a spectator approached and asked if I was okay. I offered a quick, "I'm fine, thanks," and got to my feet, just as I had after being knocked backward off my bike in college. I walked for a few minutes, thankfully in the right direction, then alternated running (shuffling, really) and walking for the next four-plus hours. When I ran each of the two laps through town, Melissa was jumping up and down, cheering and waving a sign for me. Kevin and his girlfriend, Grace, were there, too. I whimpered to Kevin, "I can't believe I have three more hours left."

"You look great!" he said, smiling.

My biggest fear had been not biking fast enough to reach the cutoff in time. That fear went unrealized and was replaced midrace with the notion that I might drop dead of exhaustion like Pheidippides after he ran from Marathon to Athens around 500 BC. But at 9:00 p.m., I finished the race and officially became an Ironman. Melissa gave me a huge hug and kiss. I stumbled under the weight of her embrace. "I'm so proud of you," Kevin told me as he patted my back. My marathon time was nearly as long as my bike time, a dubious distinction in the world of triathlon. Nearly 20 percent of the entrants failed to finish—a record for any Ironman event at that time. It was the single toughest physical endeavor of my life, and I was elated.

I woke up the next morning feeling as if nothing had happened—perhaps because I walked half the marathon or because of my euphoria from finishing—or possibly it had all been a dream. While Melissa was still asleep in the hotel bed, as tired from cheering for fifteen hours as I was from racing, I went to the bathroom and peed, realizing it was the first time I had urinated since the swim the day before. With that level of dehydration, I was lucky not to have suffered heat stroke or rhabdomyolysis, a critical condition in which muscle fibers rapidly break down and release proteins into the bloodstream. Despite my sense of accomplishment, I vowed to *never* do another Ironman again.

Melissa could not have been more supportive. The money I spent on the bike and the race. The time I spent training. My bike setup for workouts in the living room for months on end. Her nonstop cheering on race day. Our celebration with beers at a Cubs game a few days later. I was so lucky to have her.

Two months after that, Melissa got pregnant. I finished my residency the following summer, and Melissa quit her beloved job as lead transplant coordinator. I accepted a sports medicine fellowship, and we bid goodbye to Chicago, the place where we had met. I was sad to leave Kevin, but he was in a good place, and I felt assured he would stay sober.

When I started my fellowship at Massachusetts General Hospital, I was as eager as I could be. This was Harvard, after all. I would be working under the head team physicians for the New England Patriots, Boston Red Sox, Boston Bruins, and New England Revolution. I began under the tutelage of the former head team physician for the Patriots, Dr. Arturs Ozolins. An older surgeon, he was the head team physician for decades until he had been usurped by his younger protégé, who took over the leading role by clearly demonstrating his dedication to the team and surgical skills on injured players. Ozolins accepted his new role as lieutenant with grace.

It had been two years since the change in command when I got to Boston. The pecking order had been firmly established by that time. My first impression of both surgeons was that they were very focused and intense. I was scolded on my first day by Dr. Ozolins for chewing gum, then on my second day for asking a question during surgery. A necktie was compulsory at all times at the hospital unless we were operating. That included when entering the building from the parking lot, even if we were to be operating the remainder of the day. While this buttoned-up approach was a little more serious than what I had experienced at Northwestern, the care of the patients was equally meticulous at both hospitals.

I realized very early on that Dr. Ozolins did surgeries in a way I had not seen before. He likened his traditional techniques to that of a sculptor. While I could appreciate the art and skill of his approach, I could not reconcile why he wouldn't embrace the increased efficiency and precision of less archaic methods. I wondered how this man could have been the head team physician for an organization as reputable as the New England Patriots for so long, but his professional approach to everything spoke volumes.

In contrast, Dr. Gavin was skillful, up to speed on the newest surgical techniques, and relatively young. He had boundless energy, the likes of which I had never seen. He would see patients or operate all day, then cover baseball games or football practices in the evenings. He even found time to play squash in the morning before work. I had no experience with anyone who could juggle as many responsibilities as Dr.

Gavin. He would take phone calls in the middle of surgery from the Patriots' head trainer, who was demanding updates on multiple players on behalf of the coach. Nothing rattled him, not even Coach Belichick.

Just a week before my fellowship started, we moved in with my wife's parents. We showed up with scant personal belongings, including a couple of small pieces of furniture, boxes of clothes, and kitchenware, but no car. Our Honda Accord had been stolen from the street in front of our apartment in Chicago just two weeks before we moved. I walked outside one day and spent a good hour wondering where I parked it before giving up and reporting it to the police.

As I drove our U-Haul through the state of New York en route to Boston, I got a phone call from our insurance company stating that the cops had found my car abandoned in another part of the city. I just had to come back to Chicago and get it. I pleaded with them to ship it to me, but they told me it was my responsibility to get it to New England. Until my brother graciously drove the car to Boston for me, I borrowed my in-laws' garaged Jaguar.

My wife's mother, Elena, and father, Cesidio—or "Joe" as his friends know him—grew up in Italy. They were poor in the way that only people in the old country know about. For my father-in-law, that meant no electricity, no running water, and a bed made of hay in a cold stone farmhouse. He was born to a forty-seven-year-old mother as the Allied troops' bombs were dropping around their village during World War II.

Joe and Elena moved to America in their teenage years and met in Newton, Massachusetts. They worked tirelessly to put their two daughters through a private school education and then college. When they realized they had financial security, they bought a Jaguar—which they cherished but were reluctant to drive. Perhaps it was too fancy for them. I put more miles on it the year we lived with them than they had since they bought it. They seemed to get more joy out of letting me drive it than they did driving it themselves. Still, it represented their success in the New World.

Moving in with them was a challenge for me at first. I was not used to living under someone else's roof. In many ways, though, it was one of the best years of our marriage. I grew increasingly close to my in-laws, who treated me like a king. They were generous, supportive, and proud to have a son-in-law working as a doctor at Harvard, plus happy to have their daughter back home. We were thrilled to hear them tell the stories of their childhoods in Italy, the difficult weeks they spent on the boats getting across the Atlantic, and their new lives in America, initially under the presidencies of Eisenhower and Kennedy.

Melissa was due to have our first child just four weeks after we moved in, a day before my thirty-fourth birthday in late August. Melissa's ultrasounds in Chicago had shown that the baby was small for gestational age and that there was a low amount of amniotic fluid. We were concerned, but not panicked.

We met a new obstetrician in Boston and planned to have the baby at Brigham and Women's Hospital, another of the Harvard hospitals in Boston. The ultrasound from Melissa's first visit in Boston suggested slowing of the baby's heart rate, so Melissa's doctor told us they should induce her and deliver the baby then and there. Melissa burst into tears. "But I'm not ready!" she said.

"But you're nine months pregnant! When do you think you'll be ready?" I asked.

"Let's just wait one more day," she pleaded, tears still flowing.

The obstetrician agreed that this was not emergent and would contact us the next day.

That night Melissa began to have contractions, one week shy of her due date. She let me sleep through the night and then told me when I awoke that she'd been having contractions for the past six hours.

We went to the hospital, and Melissa was told that her cervix was not yet dilated, indicating she was not very far along in labor. The obstetrician on call, a woman we had never met, advised us to go home and come back later when the contractions were closer together. But Melissa was having none of it. She protested, and ultimately the OB relented.

After Melissa was admitted, she continued to contract with advancing pain. But she was still not dilated, so the OB tried to dilate her cervix manually. Melissa wailed. She still didn't dilate much. The anesthesiologist told her she would have to wait to get an epidural or else it would slow her labor. Again, she protested, convincingly enough that she got the epidural and immediately became a far more rational, peaceful person.

Once Melissa was settled in, she was put on a fetal heart rate monitor. Yet another new obstetrician came in and introduced herself as Dr. Gonzalez. She was a focused woman with soulful eyes and expressed some concern about decelerations in the fetal heart rate, showing Melissa how to change positions if the monitor's alarms went off. For the next several hours the alarms sounded periodically, prompting the nurses to come check on Melissa and the baby to make sure everything was okay, moving her from side to side to increase the baby's heart rate.

After darkness fell, we lay down until I fell asleep, Melissa dozing intermittently between contractions. At 11:30 p.m., the alarms began to ring again. Melissa woke and hoped they would stop without the nurses coming in. She was exhausted from the long labor and the lack of sleep the night before. Moments later, I was startled awake as the nurses burst into the room and turned on all the lights. Dr. Gonzalez followed and quickly moved Melissa on her hands and knees to try to get the baby's heart rate up. The monitor showed a steady deceleration that would not break.

After more than a minute, Dr. Gonzalez calmly commanded, "Get the OR ready."

"Wait," Melissa said, looking up at her with worried eyes. "What's going on?"

"We have to get the baby out. The heart rate is down, and it's not coming back up."

Melissa began to tear up. I stood there in disbelief. I was used to being the doctor, not the patient or family member.

Off Melissa went to the operating room just a few doors away. I was given surgical scrubs to change into, followed by instructions as though I had never been in an operating room before. As far as they knew, I hadn't. I was told to sit in a chair outside the OR and asked to wait for someone to come get me. The next ten minutes seemed like an eternity. What the hell could be taking so long?

When they finally came, I was shaking with anxiety. Melissa was on the operating room table, and Dr. Gonzalez was standing beside her, about to make an incision. As the scalpel was pulled across her skin, Melissa howled. The epidural was not covering her pain.

"I don't care about the pain," Melissa said. "Just cut me open."

Ignoring her pleas, the anesthesiologist dosed her with more anesthetic, and Dr. Gonzalez waited a minute before proceeding. As Dr. Gonzales worked quickly, Melissa began to panic. The epidural was working its way up her spinal column and making her suddenly feel like she was suffocating.

"I can't breathe. I can't breathe," she repeated as tears streamed down the side of her face toward the operating room table. I held her hand and put my forehead against her face.

"It's okay. You're going to be okay," I said.

"You're smothering me!" she yelped.

I sat back up and stroked her head. Instantly the baby was out. "It's a boy," Dr. Gonzalez stated jovially.

Then . . . silence.

I looked over at our baby boy. He was blue like a Smurf and covered in dark blood. After a few interminable moments, he let out a tiny whimper and then a legitimate cry. He started to pink up. As worried as I had been about the low amniotic fluid and as freaked out as I was about the night's events, that cry told me everything was going to be all right. Something deep inside me knew our new baby boy was going to be okay.

As Melissa had her incision sewn closed, they asked me to come see our son across the room under the radiant warmer that made him look like a fast-food item under a heat lamp.

"Is he normal? Is he normal?" Melissa repeatedly asked me.

"He's perfect," I reassured her. "Everything is going to be okay."

We got back to the room around 12:30 a.m. and tried our best to get some rest. Melissa attempted to feed the baby periodically when the nurses brought him in. At 7:00 a.m., I called work and let Dr. Ozolins's secretary know that I would not be in that day because we had just had a baby.

This call was followed promptly by another call, this time from Dr. Ozolins to my cell phone. He informed me that he needed me in the office and that a father's responsibility was to go to work. I told him I was not coming in, to which he responded, "We will see you at noon."

I was furious. I was not an intern anymore. I had been through the trenches for years, and my status as a fellow should have afforded me some discretion. Thirty minutes later I was called by my fellowship director, to whom Dr. Ozolins had reported my insubordination. I told him I wasn't coming in. He told me he expected me to be there the next day and hung up. I was supposed to be enjoying the birth of my son and looking after my wife, but instead I was beside myself with anger and disbelief. I wanted to quit. I could go into practice without a fellowship. I had been taught by the best in Chicago; did I really need this extra year?

I tried my best to forget about the unpleasant interactions with the two men I would spend the next year of my life learning from and serving. I focused on Melissa and trying to name our new child. Later that night, exhausted and delirious from a long labor and a narcotic pain pill she was given, Melissa could barely sit upright. The pain medication or the epidural had given her a terrible headache. With Melissa's eyes half closed and her body slumping over, I held her breast and the nurse held the baby as we tried to get him some milk. It was nearly as comical as it was concerning.

In the end, we named our son Owen, I went to work the next day, and Melissa sobered up. She and Owen went home on hospital day five, and I stuck with my fellowship. I'm so thankful I did.

MY EXPERIENCE HELPING COVER THE NEW ENGLAND Patriots was, in many ways, the highlight of my career. It seemed like a reward for all those years of hard work. While I may have been merely an assistant to the team doctor, it was a great honor. My first time at Gillette Stadium, I called the head trainer to let him know I was there. Some thirty minutes later, he walked me to security to get my photo taken and my badge made, officially christening me as part of the team.

The badge read:

GILLETTE STADIUM

MICHAEL GALLAGHER

TEAM DOCTOR

It had a giant red P next to my photo and the logo for the Patriots and the Revolution at the bottom. This would let me in the locked doors of the stadium and get me past the security guards on game days.

I was shown through the locker room, then into the training room. The locker room was bigger than it looked on TV and had a supernatural quality that I couldn't quite put my finger on. The team physician's office was a few feet beyond the double doors to the right of Tom Brady's locker, sitting just inside the training room with a desk, an exam table, X-ray light boxes, and a private bathroom. More than three or four people would make the room feel very crowded.

There were two other sports medicine fellows with me that year. Together, we covered practices both outside on the fields behind the stadium and occasionally in the inflatable indoor bubble.

I've always been curious about what goes on behind the curtain. I want to know how things work. Being with the Patriots scratched that itch for me. I was privy to the operations of the most successful franchise in NFL history.

I met Tom Brady, Bill Belichick, and Robert Kraft along with scores of other famous players, including Tedy Bruschi and Junior Seau, though not a single one of them could remember me if you pointed a gun at their head. I am one of hundreds of people who have been through that organization. For the most part, they act the same way at the stadium as they do in interviews. Bill Belichick is a prime example of that.

After one particular surgery on an injured player, Coach Belichick and Mr. Kraft came into the team doctor's office, where I was standing beside Dr. Gavin. I was taken aback for a moment seeing them both walk into the office together. The room felt nanoscopic in that moment. "How did the surgery go?" Belichick asked.

Dr. Gavin glibly responded, "Perfect," not offering any more than that. He had answered this question before.

"You fucking doctors," Belichick retorted. "Seven thousand surgeries and seven thousand of them went perfect!"

Gavin smiled wryly. "Seven thousand and one, Coach."

It was but a brief conversation that neither of them probably remember, but it represented so much of what my time with the Patriots was like. Excellence was the only option there.

EARLY ON IN MY FELLOWSHIP, I BEGAN TO LOOK FOR A job. I was anxious to get back to Colorado or somewhere else out west if possible. I felt the mountains were calling me. I did not find many job listings out there, though, so I sent a cold inquiry to a practice in Bozeman, Montana, a town I had never been to. I was delighted when they expressed interest. I flew out there for an initial interview and felt the job would be a great fit. I'd be covering college sports for Montana State University and the local ski mountain, Bridger Bowl. When I was invited back for a second interview, I brought Melissa with me. The senior partner in the group drove us to dinner the evening of the interview. While driving, he received a call from one of the other partners. We could overhear the conversation. They were going to offer me the job at dinner.

And they did. I wanted to stand up and say, "Absolutely. I will take it." After all, this practice was the only group in town, they were making an absolute killing, and they enjoyed as much as twelve weeks of vacation each year. But I knew Melissa had reservations. She was concerned that this incredibly busy group would require a huge time commitment from me, given the sports coverage. She also feared being home alone as a new mother, rarely seeing me and living in a town far from her family where she knew no one. I worried about that, too. So I responded, "Thank you very much. That is a great offer. Melissa and I will have something wonderful to discuss when we get home."

The table went dead silent. Clearly they had expected me to accept the offer on the spot.

Melissa and I ultimately decided that she would be unhappy in Montana. So I turned down the job. Secretly, though, I wished it would somehow work out in the future.

That fall, I interviewed with several other orthopedic surgery practices and accepted an offer with a very small group in Rhode Island, where I felt I would fit in best and Melissa would be happy and close to her family.

The rest of fellowship went smoothly, in part because we had no more babies that year. I was thrilled to be on the sidelines during Patriots practices and games alike, both at home and away. I flew with the team to places like Lambeau Field, where I witnessed Brady, Favre, and Rodgers all play in the same game and got to see the inner workings of the hallowed stadium. Our chartered flights were comically full of food courses, starting with snacks, then entrees, then desserts and ice cream, then gum and candies, and so on. Tray table rules and the like didn't apply. I felt like royalty. We even had police escorts lead our buses to the team hotels and the stadiums. Every bus seat was meticulously assigned, though I managed to accidentally get on the players' bus one game, not realizing it until it was too embarrassingly late to get off.

The surgeries we did over the course of the year were very similar and often identical to the ones I had learned at Northwestern. I was getting the hang of operating with more and more independence, and part of me felt like I just needed to go out and be on my own. Before finishing fellowship, I spent three months with another surgeon who was well known in the academic world of shoulder surgery. He lived up to his reputation of having a large ego, but it worked to the fellows' advantage. He loved to hear himself talk, so he was constantly teaching us.

The surgeon had his own shoulder fellowship that intertwined with my sports medicine fellowship. The shoulder fellow on service with me at the time was a Lebanese surgeon named Bassem, who had completed a hand surgery fellowship the year before at the Mayo Clinic. He was at MGH for a year of shoulder surgery, in hopes of creating an academic practice that would address upper extremity paralysis from issues such as nerve injuries.

Bassem had been a resident one year ahead of me in Chicago across town at the University of Illinois Chicago. While at UIC, Bassem made a reputation for himself as a brilliant, ambitious resident. Residents from Northwestern who had worked with Bassem at Cook County Hospital, where our programs overlapped, spoke as highly of him as I had ever heard them speak of anyone. To me he was a mythological resident, a mix of James Bond and Tony Stark.

When I finally met Bassem in Boston, he exceeded his reputation. He was whip-smart and could quote the medical literature of both hand and shoulder surgery. He spoke on the level of our attending, who was twenty-five years further into an academic career. His surgical skills exceeded those of most of the attendings. To boot, Bassem was incredibly nice, calm, and confident.

He charmed patients with his Middle Eastern accent and his constant guessing of their astrological signs. "You seem very enthusiastic. I am sure you must be an Aries. Am I correct?" he would ask. At times, he seemed as interested in patients' birth months as he was in their shoulder problems. Operating with Bassem was an incredible lesson in just how important confidence is as a surgeon.

THE END OF MY FELLOWSHIP WAS MARRED BY THE DEATH of Melissa's grandmother, Caterina Serra, or Nonina to all the grandchildren. Melissa had been incredibly close to Nonina, and she was one of the reasons we stayed near Boston. When Nonina got sick, Melissa spent every moment she could taking care of her. She died just a month after the family found out she had cancer that had spread to her organs. At ninety-four years of age, she was still on her feet cooking all day. She lived on the second floor of a house owned by one of her daughters. She still carried fifty-pound bags of flour up the stairs herself. After more than forty years of living in the United States, she spoke very few words in English, adding to her charm. At age eighty, she had been forced into retirement from her job at a local factory.

She was tough, in part because she had it tough.

In Italy, she had a difficult life with an alcoholic husband, the family barely making ends meet by farming. She lost her only son, her firstborn child, when the bassinet holding him fell over, causing him to suffocate. The police threatened to file charges, but never did. Around 1960, she moved to the United States with her husband and three teenage daughters. She became the matriarch of the family and brought with her all the Italian traditions her ancestors handed down — including many Melissa would carry on.

I wouldn't know just how hard Melissa took her grandmother's death until we moved to Rhode Island.

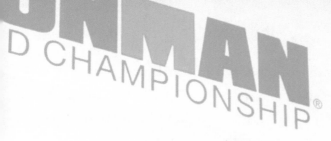

Chapter 7

It's Just My Stomach

I finished fellowship eager to start my career. We would be moving just an hour and a half away to southern Rhode Island. The town of South Kingstown sits just across the Narragansett Bay from opulent Newport, famous for its extraordinary mansions. We would be living in the village of Wakefield, a pastoral hamlet heavily thicketed and strewn with sod farms. Hand-built, seemingly ancient stone walls lined the narrow country roads that meandered through the rolling hills down to the ocean.

I had a month off between the end of my fellowship and the start of my new practice in South Kingstown. Just a few months before finishing fellowship, I won a lottery spot to participate in the Ironman World Championship in Kona, Hawai'i. My vow to never race another Ironman again evaporated just a month after crossing the finish line in

Wisconsin. I began training whenever I could find time between finishing fellowship, covering Patriots practices, and taking care of Owen while Melissa was with her grandmother. Once my fellowship ended, I wanted to get in as many miles on the bike as I could, trying to avoid a repeat of my dismal performance during my first few triathlons.

I bought a new road bike, loaded it up with twenty-five pounds of gear and maps then set out from Newton bound for Maine. I would ride approximately one hundred miles each day and find a town on the map where I hoped to get a motel room. The first day the bike felt incredibly heavy as I slowly turned the pedals. I packed as light as possible, planning on wearing the same clothes every day, yet the load noticeably slowed me.

As evening approached, I pedaled into Portsmouth, New Hampshire, where I found a quaint little motel for lodging. Melissa drove up from Newton, and we spent what felt like the first night alone in months. It was heavenly for both of us. After a peaceful night's sleep free from any parenting duties or worries about work, we enjoyed a few tranquil moments reconnecting with each other, drinking coffee, and talking about our imminent life in Rhode Island and how scary the Hawai'i Ironman sounded. We held a long embrace, then Melissa drove back home in time to feed Owen, and I headed north, making my way another hundred gratifying miles up the coast along two-lane roads.

On the third day, I cut inland heading west across the idyllic countryside of Maine through towns like Buckfield, founded in 1793, population 1,723. By day four, my legs felt a compulsion to pedal as if being commanded by a higher power. It was unlike anything I'd ever felt. I was starting to gain confidence that I could be strong on the bike for the duration of the Ironman in Hawai'i. I stayed the night in Conway, New Hampshire, and then rode up over Crawford Notch, past Bretton Woods, site of a ski area and the Mount Washington Hotel, which hosted a famous delegation during World War II that established the International Monetary Fund and the basis for international currency exchange. The hotel itself is a massive white façade speckled with windows and covered with a red roof that sits below a range of ever-clouded mountains. I continued on to the Town of Carroll, where Melissa's parents had a vacation house. I slept there one night, then rode down to Lake Winnipesaukee the next day, where Melissa met me for a quick getaway near a house her father was renovating. I practiced my open-water swimming as Melissa kayaked next to me, keeping the occasional motorboat at a safe distance.

The weeklong bike ride seemed to prepare me well for my Ironman in early October. I felt awkward asking for a week off to go to Hawai'i just five weeks after starting my new job, but this chance didn't come around very often. My new partners were gracious about letting me go. I was relatively new to Ironman racing and not nearly fast enough on the bike to qualify for Kona, so a lottery slot was the only realistic way I would ever get to race there. In medical school, I watched the annual specials on the Ironman athletes, which often told the story of lottery winners who were there not because of their amazing speed but because of some even more impressive obstacle they had overcome or a battle they were fighting—cancer, the loss of a child, even ALS. I was mesmerized by the athletes' superhuman feats, especially those of Dick Hoyt, who pulled, pedaled, and pushed his adult son, Rick, who had cerebral palsy, for all 140.6 miles.

Melissa and I arrived in Kona three days before the race. That gave me enough time to reassemble my bike, pick up my race number, familiarize myself with the course, and take in the scene around town. Lava Java, a coffee shop just south of the race start/finish, was abuzz with athletes of the fittest kind imaginable. Unlike Ironman Wisconsin and many of the marathons I'd run, everyone here looked the part. There were no beer bellies or flabby arms. I looked horribly out of place just for not having shaved legs. I was in the best shape of my life, and I didn't hold a candle to these athletes. Melissa and I slept with the air conditioning off and the windows open in hopes that I would acclimate to the heat and humidity.

In the days before the race, the roads were packed with athletes running and riding everywhere. I had always done best with plenty of rest before a race, so I resisted the temptation to go out and train amongst the others. I was saving my energy for the underpants run two days before the race, but somehow, I missed out on that salacious outing. Perhaps it was just as well that I rested because I started to feel nauseated that day. I felt sick the next day, as well. Melissa believed it was nerves, but I hadn't ever felt this way before a race. This continued through Friday, the day before the race, when I checked my bike and gear in for Saturday.

Saturday morning, I awoke at 1:30 a.m. and let out a groan that awakened Melissa. "What's wrong?" she asked.

"I'm fine," I mumbled. "It's just my stomach."

"Are you sure you are okay to race?"

I gave a specious rebuttal to prevent the conversation from going further. "I will be fine. Worst-case scenario, I can just drop out."

"You won't, though. You never have," she replied.

I got out of bed and sipped on a five-hundred-calorie protein drink until it was gone. It sat in my stomach like a brick. I lay there awake and sweaty until 4:00 a.m. and then filled my belly again with a thousand calories of oatmeal, bagels, and more protein drink. At 5:00 a.m., Melissa drove me to the start line. We picked up another athlete who was walking toward the start in the dark. She was around forty and looked fit like the masses at Lava Java. She told us that in late August, she had raced her first Ironman in Louisville, Kentucky, and qualified for Kona. Here she was doing two Ironman races in just six weeks. I couldn't imagine recovering from an Ironman and being ready to race again in so little time. I didn't get back on my bike again for six months after Wisconsin.

I got my race number marked on my arms, checked my bike setup, pumped up my tires, and left the start area to go find Melissa. We saw surfer Laird Hamilton, who was there to lead the pro swimmers on a stand-up paddleboard, and his wife, professional volleyball player and model Gabrielle Reece. I encouraged Melissa to go over and talk with Gabrielle, who was in line for coffee. Melissa was awestruck at how nice and beautiful she was. While the two were having a pleasant conversation, a team of Navy SEALS jumped out of a plane and parachuted into the water, captivating the crowd. The gun for the pros went off at 6:45 a.m. The mass start for the rest of us was to be at 7:00 a.m. sharp, the delay ensuring the professionals that their day would not be marred by any overzealous amateurs trying to swim recklessly at the front to be a part of the action.

As seven o'clock approached, most of the athletes were treading water just behind the invisible start line demarcated by a band of surfboards being paddled back and forth, holding the swimmers at bay. To avoid mass swim start troubles and conserve as much energy as possible, I loitered at the entry to the water, waiting until the last moment to get all the way in. My plan was to gently swim out to the start, staying just a bit behind the two thousand other athletes. I knew I would not be as fast as most of these athletes, especially those in my age group.

But when the gun went off, I was still in waist-deep water 150 yards from the start. I had miscalculated the time. The gun startled me, and I dove forward. By the time I got up to the crowd of swimmers, I realized I was stuck behind the slowest bunch.

I swam steadily until I got to a group going the same speed as me. Because the ocean water in Kona is consistently close to eighty degrees, no wetsuits are allowed—which made for a slower swim for athletes like me who had little body fat to lend buoyancy. I still had my sights on a swim around one hour and ten minutes, though. As we got farther out in Kailua Bay and I ingested more and more briny water, my nausea began to return. Staring through slightly fogged goggles into a solid blue abyss worsened the situation. I tried to stay calm and keep pace, eventually making it back to the pier ten minutes past my goal. I heard the announcer call my name as I raced out of the water, up the staircase onto the pier, and into the makeshift transition area, where I threw on my triathlon top and slathered sunblock all over my face, neck, arms, and legs. As I exited the changing tent, I noticed just how few bikes were left on the pier. Those remaining were way up front near the exit, indicating they belonged to the oldest age groups—those over sixty. I was in a different league for sure.

The stories about the heat and wind in Kona are legendary. The NBC coverage talks about it every year. The winds tend to blow moderately hard on the first half of the bike ride and intensify as the day warms during the second half. That's if you're fast. For slower bikers like me, it means the winds are going to howl for seventy or eighty miles.

The first several miles on the bike I felt wretched. I was pedaling hard, but my bike computer was telling me I was barely moving along. Despite this, I was passing a few people. I downed an entire bottle of water in the first twenty minutes, then started to feel better. Once my stomach issues abated, I felt great and it was easygoing for a couple of hours until the fifteen-mile climb up the mountain to the town of Hawi. The last five miles up to the turnaround point the heat and winds noticeably intensified, but I made steady progress.

I got to Hawi feeling good. Sixty miles down and fifty-two miles to go. I was on track to ride six hours and thirty minutes, which was great if I wanted to break twelve hours, an admirable goal for a lottery winner. I stopped to get extra food at the turnaround and use the bathroom quickly and then was rewarded with a fifteen-mile downhill. But then Madame Pele had her fun with me as I quickly learned exactly what makes Kona Kona. Whether it was from not eating enough calories or the onset of the steady headwind, I do not know, but my bike speed plummeted, dashing my time goal for the bike. For the last twenty-two miles, the winds were crushing me and the few cyclists left around me.

I made it back to town and quickly put my running shoes on with no doubt that I would continue on. Clouds rolled in off the sea just as I started the run, which was a welcomed relief from the intense sun I had experienced so far. At mile four, I saw Melissa jumping up and down, screaming wildly for me. I stopped and said hello, then gave her a kiss, telling her I would see her again after reaching the run turnaround a few miles away.

I resolved to run at least the first thirteen miles without stopping, but somewhere around mile eleven, my stomach started killing me again. I ate some bread to try to stem the hunger and stomach pain and then started alternating walking and running. Eventually, the pain became so intense that I simply could not run anymore. I became nervous not only about finishing but also about my GI tract.

I walked down the hill into the notoriously hot Natural Energy Lab just as the sun disappeared from the sky around 6:00 p.m. My special needs bag was down there, and I desperately wanted my albuterol inhaler. At that point, though, it was my stomach that was the real problem. As I left the lab, an electronic sign that read my electronic chip flashed 1272 MICHAEL GALLAGHER—ALMOST THERE. Another runner urged me to go with him to the finish line, but I just couldn't run anymore. Every attempt to run increased the stabbing pain in my abdomen. I walked at a pace that was fast enough to get me to the finish before midnight, but not double me over with belly pain. I was riding a fine line. I worried each moment that the next step would be my last.

With less than a mile to go, I turned onto Ali'i Drive, home of Ironman's famous finish line and the most coveted prize in all of triathlon. That's when I started to run. A shuffle at first, and then it built into a true run and eventually a sprint. As I neared the finish line, I saw Melissa through the blinding lights. The announcer, Mike Riley, was calling my name. People on the bleachers were high-fiving me. I ran up a ramp as fast as I could, raised my arms to the sky, and crossed the finish line in thirteen hours and forty-one minutes. I was grinning ear to ear.

A flower lei was put around my neck and an Ironman towel was thrown on my shoulders. Two female volunteers whisked me away, congratulating me and asking me how I felt and what I needed. I thought about going to get an IV and having my belly checked, but instead I went straight for the pizza. It was the most delicious pizza of my life. And it was free—if you don't count the $450 entry fee and 140.6 miles of swimming, biking, and running required to get it.

I left Kona with a couple of souvenirs. In addition to the finisher's medal I coveted, I had a stripe of sunburn on my right thigh where my triathlon shorts crept up during the race. I looked like I had been touched with a hot branding iron. When the sunburn finally peeled a week later, it left a darkened stripe that stayed on my skin for two years—a badge of honor in my mind. As with my first Ironman, I swore I would never do another again. I was wrong again. I went on to finish one more in 2013 at Ironman Florida. Unlike Wisconsin and Hawai'i, though, in Florida I swore *before* the race that it would be my last Ironman. It turns out I was right.

Chapter 8

I Can't Stay Here

Once the distractions of moving and the Ironman abated, Melissa found herself at home with a one-year-old in a town that offered very little entertainment. Then she got pregnant again, and things seemed to change.

"I can't stay here," Melissa told me one night in November over a pasta dinner she had made by hand.

"What are you talking about? This house?" I asked, worried.

"No," she said. "Rhode Island. I hate it here."

I was stunned. "We just got here. How can you hate it already? You said you liked it when we decided to take this job."

"I don't care. I am not staying here. This place will be the death of me."

I paused. "Let's just give it a little more time."

"No amount of time will make me change my mind," she stated firmly.

"What am I supposed to do? I just started this job. How am I going to find another one?"

I had seen Melissa resolute in her decisions before. Melissa lamented that unlike the summer when things were bustling, as soon as Labor Day was over, the town was deserted. She never saw or talked to anyone but me when I got home from work. The loss of her grandmother added to her feeling of isolation and sadness.

Our time together in Rhode Island was fleeting. I was disappointed. I liked Rhode Island. I liked my practice. I loved the beautiful, rural setting.

But I loved my wife more.

After some more back-and-forth, I caved in. "Okay, I'll start looking for a new job."

We discussed what would make her happy. She said Chicago or Boston. I balked. I had no desire to live back in Chicago or practice in the shadow of Mass General. I liked living rurally. But Melissa wanted the excitement of a city. With her grandmother gone, she no longer felt the need to be in New England.

We considered college towns like Madison, Wisconsin, and Boulder, Colorado. Melissa had been to Boulder once before and loved it. It was her first choice of a new place to live. I had tried to apply for jobs in Colorado a year prior and didn't find what I was looking for. In fact, Boulder was an oversaturated market, and it was nearly impossible to establish a practice there. Fortuitously, Kaiser Permanente posted a new position in Denver right as Melissa declared her desire to leave Rhode Island. I was cautiously optimistic. Perhaps Melissa would be happy in Denver, or I could commute from Boulder. So without my group knowing, Melissa and I went to Denver for an interview with several people from the practice. That night, we met the chief and two other surgeons for dinner.

At the beginning of the dinner the chief told me, "The Denver position has been filled."

I was confused. "I didn't know that. Did that just happen? I thought I was here to interview for the job."

"Yes. We just got an acceptance from another candidate. But we are going to have another surgeon position available up in Boulder County, at our Lafayette campus."

My eyes lit up. "Really?"

A week later, I had a phone interview with the local chief of the Lafayette campus and told him I was interested.

"Well," he said deliberately, "there is one other candidate overseas with the military that we are trying to interview in person. His return has been delayed, but I have been holding the position for him."

"I understand," I said. "I would still love to come out and interview with you and meet the partners up there."

He agreed to have me out, and I interviewed with what seemed like a very nice and young group of surgeons. Jeff, the chief, was a West Point graduate and had a full military career before coming to Kaiser. That partly explained his affinity for the other candidate. He looked carefully at my résumé while interviewing me and said, "You must know the other candidate. He was a year or two ahead of you at Northwestern."

He told me the name, and I nearly choked on the water I was drinking. The guy he was talking about was one of the few people I would go out on a limb to say, "Do not ever hire this person." He had been in fistfights while out drinking, had been an asshole to me, and was an all-around bad egg. But I kept my mouth shut and didn't say a word other than, "Wow, what a coincidence."

A couple of weeks after my interview, I was offered the job and accepted. Apparently the other candidate wanted to be in a bigger city. I returned to Rhode Island and told my partners that I was leaving. They were extremely gracious and understanding. I think they could tell I was delighted working with them but that Melissa wasn't happy there.

Despite my keenness to live in Boulder again, I had some reservations about taking the job. I was told it would be 50 percent sports medicine, which was my specialty, and 50 percent trauma, which certainly was not. I did not have a trauma-heavy experience at Northwestern or Harvard. But I took a leap of faith that I would be able to rise to the occasion. Besides, I had no better option.

We stayed in Rhode Island for six more months—the time it took to get a medical license and hospital privileges in another state. I continued to see a wide variety of illnesses and injuries, including Lyme disease. Lyme disease, which is common in New England, is transmitted to humans via the bite of an infected tick. Specifically, a tiny bacterium called *Borrelia burgdorferi* causes the infection. People often notice a bull's-eye-shaped red rash surrounding the bite and develop acute symptoms such as fever, malaise, and fatigue. The infection, especially if untreated, can spread to other parts of the body, including the heart, the nervous system, and the joints. Early treatment with antibiotics is quite successful, but if treatment is delayed or never undertaken, the disease can cause devastating, chronic problems. While it is difficult to know the exact number, some studies report false negative test rates at 20 to 30 percent. As a result, Lyme disease is often missed. And the symptoms are often attributed to other conditions.

In my remaining time in Rhode Island, I saw a thirteen-year-old boy with sudden locking of his elbow. When I examined him, his elbow would not move more than five degrees in either direction from the flexed position he held it in. From the standpoint of an orthopedic surgeon, mechanical locking of the elbow is typically associated with a loose piece of cartilage or bone getting trapped in the joint, often as a result of trauma such as a dislocation. In some instances, adolescents can have this happen without an acute injury, but rather from overuse, such as pitching, a condition called osteochondritis dissecans (OCD). I ordered an MRI of his elbow to take a closer look. I also ordered a Lyme disease antibody test, thinking Lyme was unlikely to be the cause, but not wanting to miss anything. When the test came back positive, I treated him with antibiotics, and before the MRI was done, the boy's elbow was better. I was amazed at how convincing his exam had been that this was a mechanical problem rather than an infectious one.

I went on to treat handfuls of other patients with Lyme who also experienced joint pain, and not long after I saw the boy with the locked elbow, our son, Owen, who was two years old at the time, started telling us his knees hurt. He then began complaining that the lights were too bright when we would lay him on his back to change his diaper. We brought him to the pediatrician and suggested that this might be Lyme disease. The pediatrician agreed and tested him, but the test was negative. He recommended against antibiotics, knowing as I did that antibiotic overuse can cause its own problems, including antibiotic resistance. Owen continued to complain for the next couple of days, so I decided to treat him myself. Within forty-eight hours of starting the antibiotics, Owen's symptoms vanished. Had we waited or not treated him, who knows what the outcome may have been. I left Rhode Island with a great appreciation for just how subtle yet powerful infections can be, a lesson I would learn again the hard way.

THE WEEK BEFORE BEGINNING MY JOB IN COLORADO, I traveled abroad to see Liam, who was living in Germany with his wife. Liam was always a blast to hang out with, but like many others in my life, he had troubles with drugs and alcohol. He had been sober on and off for years before living in Germany. When I got there, he was back to drinking.

We went out to one of the public beer gardens early one day and caught up on each other's lives. Then we hopped around town and caught the train out to the soccer stadium for a game, but the tickets were sold out. Liam was disappointed but not deterred. He quickly came up with plan B.

"Let's go to a brothel," he said.

"What?" I asked incredulously.

"They're totally legal here. The wives drop their husbands off at these places," he stated.

"That seems far-fetched," I said.

"I'm serious. Let's just go inside. You'll get a kick out of it."

"Fine. But I'm not sleeping with any prostitute," I insisted.

Once inside, we were directed to a locker room, where we changed into towels. I was nervous about what we were in for. We passed through another door and were immediately in a bar. I felt naked. The bar was all but empty. Liam and I sat on a couple of stools and ordered a few beers.

In an adjacent room, women sauntered about topless, acting as if there was an invisible barrier between us and them. Liam disappeared for fifteen minutes or so, and I sat there alone eating what I can only assume was the filthiest bowl of peanuts in all of Germany. As I sat and drank my beer, a group of soccer fans came in hooting and hollering, also clad in nothing but towels. When Liam returned, we finished our beers and I suggested we get the hell out of there. I wasn't sure if what I had witnessed was truly the German way or just for those who got carried away.

Kevin met us the next day on a business trip. He laughed at our story from the night before, shaking his head as we regaled him with the ridiculous details. It would be the last time the three of us would get together. Not long after that, Liam's unscrupulous behavior got him in trouble at work. He lost his job and developed severe paranoid delusions that landed him back in the United States, estranged from his wife and young daughter. Eventually he was declared incompetent to stand trial for multiple criminal offenses stemming from his deranged thoughts. While everyone who loved him could easily see his struggles with drugs and alcohol, no one anticipated the onset of profound mental illness at the unusually late age of thirty-seven. The Liam we grew up with was gone for good.

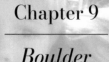

Chapter 9

Boulder

Melissa and I rented a house in downtown Boulder just off Pearl Street, the pedestrian mall that bisects the mixed upscale and bohemian downtown shopping district. We were excited to be in Boulder at last. Owen and Reese were peanuts still, far too young to remember their lives in Massachusetts or Rhode Island. They would grow up Colorado kids.

My career with Kaiser started smoothly. Jeff, the chief of our department and the man who hired me, would be my closest working partner. He and I split the management of the lion's share of the orthopedic trauma. Jeff's experience of more than twenty years was invaluable to me and to the department. Together, he and I ran our Acute Orthopedic Clinic four days a week. The remaining day was dedicated solely to hand trauma and run by one of the three hand surgeons in the group.

Jeff believed in me from the get-go. I had more expertise than he did in shoulder trauma from my fellowship at Mass General. As a result, he routinely routed a lot of the complex shoulder fractures to me and taught me his techniques for other surgeries he had more experience doing. We operated together on the most difficult cases. He trusted me with the rest.

We were an odd couple of sorts. He was a West Point graduate, experienced, quiet, and conservative. I was green both from a surgical experience and an environmentally conscious standpoint. I leaned as far left politically as he did right. But none of that mattered. We developed an immense respect for each other.

When my confidence was shaken early on, I went to Jeff and asked if he had any issues with my performance.

"I'll tell you if I do." That was all he said, and that was all I needed to hear.

Jeff was the consummate professional. He was the one to stay late for an add-on case or come in on his day off to do surgeries that others were nervous about or too inexperienced to do. He led by example. And I followed in his footsteps, trying to do as many trauma cases as possible for the sake of the patients and my partners.

In addition to teaching me clinical skills, he showed me how to be a leader. He groomed me to replace him as the chief of the department and turned the reins over to me a few years before he retired, ensuring he was there to help me along. While I had a very different style because of my personality, I held myself to the same high standards.

My other partners at Kaiser were fantastic, as well. Not every personality was the same, but the patient care was excellent—far better than I saw elsewhere in training and private practice.

Early on at Kaiser, one of my partners, Lance, asked me repeatedly to join him out for beers. I always had some reason that I couldn't—usually related to running. Thankfully, Lance was not deterred by my refusals, and eventually we got together. We soon realized we had a common fondness for mountain biking, skiing, time away from work, and irreverent humor. Lance turned out to be far more fascinating than he'd let on. He grew up one of twelve children in Hanover, Pennsylvania, and married a woman who grew up one of nine. He put himself through college and medical school, defying the odds by a long shot that he would even get out of Hanover.

Lance lived up in the foothills behind Boulder on a thirty-acre property crisscrossed by single-track mountain bike trails he created. Always in search of fun, he built a dirt racetrack for go-carts behind his house, bought a full arsenal of paintball guns and protective gear, had an endless supply of mountain bikes, and put a huge deck on the house with a hot tub and a firepit. From his house in Steamboat, he took us backcountry skiing in deep powder on snowmobiles up and down Buff Pass. He spoiled all his friends, constantly buying meals out and rounds of beers. He regaled my kids with treats and presents, even hosting their birthday parties at his house.

Colleagues like Lance and my career at Kaiser taught me to be a better surgeon. We rarely referred surgical cases outside of our own group of doctors, so we had to take care of almost everything ourselves. For me, that meant having to deal with trauma I was intimated by. So I decided from the start to tackle my fears head-on. Surgical videos, which were nonexistent when I was in training, started populating the internet, allowing me to continuously update and perfect my surgical techniques and take on more problems than I previously thought I was capable of. In many cases, I found that the widespread trepidation surrounding some surgical approaches was not warranted—it was simply a matter of unfamiliarity coupled with fearmongering that led to groupthink.

What I was not properly trained to handle was the emotional toll complications took on me. Early in my career, any complication, no matter how large or small, kept me awake at night and haunted my dreams. I could not deal with someone being worse off because of my surgery. The complications were infrequent, but the failures stick with you far more than the victories or successes.

One complication early in my career devastated me. I had a teenage patient with a shoulder that dislocated repeatedly. An MRI showed that he had a torn labrum (cartilage). The standard of care is to repair the labrum, which tightens up the ligaments, thus stabilizing the shoulder. The surgery can be done open (the older method) or arthroscopically (the currently preferred method for most cases). I performed an arthroscopic stabilization, which took no more than an hour.

Six weeks later, I saw the patient for a routine post-op visit. I noticed that his hand muscles had atrophied slightly and that two of his fingers were numb. I suspected the sling was pressing on a nerve in his elbow, so I discontinued the sling, which he was due for anyway. But a month later, the atrophy was worse. I sent him for a nerve study that suggested an injury to the nerves just above his shoulder. The disability in his hand would be permanent.

I immediately blamed myself and tried to make sense of what had happened. I suspected a nerve block he'd had before surgery caused his nerve damage, but I could not shake the worry that it was from the surgery itself. When I saw the patient and his mother back in the office, I wept. Would his life be the same? Did he regret ever meeting me?

"I am so deeply sorry," I said. They didn't know what to say in return but handled my apology graciously. I saw him over the course of the following year and then never again.

I was anxious about this type of surgery for a while after that case. I doubted myself. Eventually, I realized that even if his nerve injury was a direct result of my surgery, I could not undo it. I did my best and offered a heartfelt apology, which allowed me to stop blaming myself, but it never completely left me.

As the years progressed, I developed what I felt were excellent surgical skills, allowing me to approach my cases full of confidence but not arrogance. I left the OR feeling proud of my performance. There was very little I feared anymore. At least not at work.

When I got sick in 2014 on the Maah Daah Hey Trail in North Dakota, I feared I might never race another marathon again. Then that I might never run at all. Then that I might never work again.

Then that I might not survive another day.

Chapter 10

The Badlands

The Badlands, North Dakota, in late May 2014 was the opposite of Boston in April 2013 when the bombs went off on Boylston Street. It was hot and barren. There were no tall buildings, just short, steep, sandy hills. There were no throngs of people, just a few intrepid mountain bikers. It was the most remote place I had ever been, serene yet foreboding.

My trip to the Badlands started inauspiciously. Three days before I departed, I became ill with a virus—the bomb itself or perhaps an accelerant adding to the fatigue I had felt in Boston. Our neighbor across the street, a cute two-year-old named Kieran with a perfectly symmetrical round face, and his older brother played at our house every day with our son and daughter. Kieran came down with a case of Coxsackievirus, also known as hand, foot, and mouth disease

—a common illness among children. He had the classic rash associated with it, a telltale sign for pediatricians and parents alike. Atypically, his mother got it, too; the virus usually doesn't transmit to adults. Next to get sick were my wife and daughter, both of whom developed the familiar accompanying rash. Our daughter spiked fevers of 105 degrees and was miserable. Eventually, I also felt sick, and debated whether to go on my much-anticipated bike trip.

Having awaited this pilgrimage to the Badlands for years, I was reluctant to cancel for what I figured was going to be a short-lived malady. It was a reunion with guys I had spent a full week mountain biking with five years before. They called themselves the Ugly Bastards. I had pushed through illnesses many times before, including colds and GI bugs, running or biking instead of resting, never wanting to lose fitness. I always came out on the other side unscathed. So I decided to tough it out this time, too.

As we left for Medora, North Dakota, where we would embark upon the Maah Daah Hey trail, I was still feeling wretched. I reckoned that a day's drive would allow me to rest, and I'd be better by the time we started pedaling. Mark, a slightly older friend and neighbor whom I looked up to immensely, rode in the passenger seat as we drove through Wyoming in a year when the normally brown, rolling fields were as green as the hills of Ireland. It was gorgeous and for a few hours I tried to forget how sick I felt. We cut across the northwest corner of South Dakota and into southern North Dakota. As we pulled into Medora, we met up with Rod, my friend from medical school, and the rest of the Ugly Bastards, who had all driven together in a rented RV from northern California.

The inaugural Ugly Bastards trip in 2009 was for Rod's and his friend Bill's fortieth birthdays. We rode from Durango, Colorado, to Moab, Utah, for seven insanely awesome days, staying in one-room wooden huts with wood burning stoves, coolers stocked with eggs and bacon, and eight primitive bunk beds. It was the trip of a lifetime. I finished in one piece, save for a sprained ligament in my thumb. This trip with the Ugly Bastards, however, wouldn't end as well.

Maah Daah Hey, American Indian for something that has been around or will be around for a long time, is an iconic trail for mountain bikers and listed as one of the world's Epic Rides. I was excited to see the guys again. This year, mustaches were mandatory and several varieties were represented, including ones that looked like they belonged on a long haul trucker, and others that were reminiscent of a seventies porn star. It was all in good fun, but when it came to mountain biking, we were serious. The harder the day was, the more it proved we were supposed to be there. So showing up sick was not something I was ready to admit to.

The 2010 census put the population of Medora at 112. Tourism and the oil industry balloon the town at certain times of the year, but year-round residents are few. One of those people was a guy named Loren, co-owner of Dakota Cyclery and our local guide. We went to his bike store the first day we were in Medora to get supplies and discuss our itinerary with Loren. Having finished my second Boston Marathon just six weeks before, my six-feet-three, 140-pound body was made for speed and endurance, not strength or raw power. Nonetheless, I found myself on a rented, much too heavy, full-suspension Cannondale bike that I would have to muscle up and down the steep hills of the Badlands.

The following morning Loren loaded the nine of us up in his truck with all our bikes to head to the southernmost part of the trail, a new extension that looped back to Medora. Loren had strongly recommended we do this part of the ride first because the recent heavy rainfall made several parts of the Maah Daah Hey unpassable; the mud was so thick.

At the start of the trail, the conditions seemed pretty favorable. But once we were a few miles in, we realized that the sandy terrain made finding the trail difficult, so while we were spared the sticky mud that other parts of the trail were plagued by, our progress was still slowed by our need to navigate. Stopping every 15 to 20 minutes, though, gave me a chance to catch my breath. As the day progressed and the heat intensified, I realized I was in bad shape. I was feeling sick, but I kept my mouth shut and pedaled on.

Not too far in, one of the other riders, Finn, started to show signs that he, too, was ill. Each time we stopped to look at the map or scout the trail, he would take refuge on the ground. He told us he wasn't feeling well and needed to rest. This was his first trip with the Ugly Bastards. Like me, Finn was a physician, but he clearly spent more time in the gym lifting weights than he did on a bike. As my own symptoms worsened, I realized that Finn and I might be brothers-in-arms.

More than six hours after we departed, we hit a dirt road and stopped once again to look at the map. The dirt road would take us back to town and end my misery, whereas continuing on the trail would require an hour or so more of strenuous single-track biking. The rest of the Ugly Bastards opted for the trail, while Finn and I chose to bail out and take the gravel road home.

No more than five minutes after the rest of the crew left, Finn started projectile vomiting. All the water he had been drinking to try to quench his thirst and cool himself down never made it past his stomach. This was a clear sign of heat exhaustion. When the body is overheating, it will shut down digestion, sending blood to your skin instead to cool you down. That's exactly what happened that day to Finn. Being in pretty rough shape myself, I was happy to stop every so often to allow Finn to vomit or lie on the ground to recuperate.

After more than an hour of walking our bikes and stopping for rest, I noticed a thunderhead cloud in the sky west of us. This bad boy would be bearing down on us within an hour or two. Daylight was at a premium, as well. I implored Finn to try to ride, but he just couldn't do it. The slightest uphill was too much energy for him to expend. I told Finn that if he couldn't get moving, I would ride back to town, get a car, and come back to get him. Staying out there during the storm would lead to the opposite problem he was having. Hypothermia.

Finn took my advice, using all his energy to walk the uphills and coast on his bike along the downhills. As we continued to make slow progress toward Medora, a small, white, dilapidated, government-issued pickup truck came upon us, heading toward town. It was a godsend for Finn. We flagged the driver down and asked for a ride. He had but one seat in the cab, and the bed was filled with metal fenceposts and barbed wire. The driver and I put Finn's bike on top of the payload and Finn slumped into the passenger seat. I reassured him I'd meet him back in town.

As Finn closed the door, I was met out on the road by the rest of the Ugly Bastards who had emerged from the trail just minutes prior. I recapped our adventures to them as I rode with the guys the rest of the way into town, making it just before the storm cloud unleashed its fury on the Badlands.

The following morning I awoke still sick and worn out from the day before. It was a blow to my ego, but I decided I was too sick to ride. Instead, I rode in Loren's truck with a trailer full of our gear to our campsite for that night. Finn rallied and saddled up with the guys, shocking all of us and leaving me concerned he may be in for a repeat performance.

As we drove out of Medora, Loren said no more than ten words to me. We were headed west toward Montana and then would turn north toward Canada to get to the campsite. Earlier, as I rested in town, he had taken the Ugly Bastards up to their starting point northeast of Medora. They would meet us at the campsite after a six-hour ride.

On the way, Loren and I stopped by his house and then got gas in Sentinel Butte, a town just west of Medora, population ninety-one. Olsen's Service, a one-pump gas station, looked like it belonged in Mayberry, along with Andy Griffith and Barney Fife. Loren parked under the gas station awning, opened his door, turned perpendicular to the seat, and just sat there. His legs dangled out the side of the truck, his boots a foot off the dusty ground. Both of us looked at the store.

An older man eventually ambled out. "Hey."

After considering his response for a good ten seconds, Loren responded. "Hey."

That seemed to be the end of the conversation. Then after another pause, the store owner said, "So, how's it going?"

"Okay, I guess," Loren said. Twenty seconds later, he asked, "You?"

On this went, with each question and answer carefully deliberated. The entire conversation consisted of less than thirty words and took a solid three minutes.

I was mesmerized. It had been so long since I'd seen such genuine humanity and lack of pretense. It reminded me of my childhood in the days before cable TV and the internet, when human interaction was our most precious commodity.

As Loren drove the trailer full of gear and me toward our campsite, we traveled along the most remote expanse of open prairie I had ever seen. It seemed you could go forty miles between signs of life. I asked Loren about the small town where he lived and the gas station we had just been to.

He told me that the owner of the store was a friend of his, and in fact, a friend of everyone who lived in Sentinel Butte. In years past, he left the store open so anyone in town was free to come in and purchase whatever they wanted anytime they wanted. They would leave their names and what they took on the pad of paper on the counter, and he would put it on their tab.

That system was corrupted a few years back, though, when an Oprah Winfrey Show episode about honesty featured the gas station's owner. It turns out people are willing to steal from strangers quite easily. Once the show aired, people found their way off I-90 and into town, where the store sat unlocked, ready to be pilfered. The owner didn't let that stop him, though. Knowing he couldn't leave the store unlocked anymore, he gave copies of keys to the store to every family in town, allowing them to continue to use the honor system that kept the community so tight-knit.

I would later feel part of a community that tight-knit myself. There were no keys handed out in this new community I would become a part of, though. There were common experiences instead—physical and mental suffering, post-exertional malaise, disregard by the medical community, and skepticism from coworkers and friends.

After a day of rest, I rode the remainder of the Maah Daah Hey, biting my lip and pedaling through two days full of endless amounts of that thick mud Loren promised us. When I returned home, I knew something was wrong. I sensed a seismic shift in my wellbeing. It would take several dispiriting years for me to figure out what that something was. It was chronic fatigue.

Chapter 11

Run Down

When I returned home to Boulder from North Dakota in 2014, I was exhausted, still feeling the effects of the virus that crushed me on the Maah Daah Hey Trail. I took the next week and a half off from exercise to convalesce. For the past five years, I had not taken more than five consecutive days off from exercise, but this exhaustion called for drastic action.

I had returned to hard workouts way faster than I had anticipated after the Boston Marathon, six weeks before the bike trip. I considered that this might be another reason I should rest. As the days went along, the viral symptoms cleared. I planned my year ahead, anticipating that I would race the Chicago Marathon in the fall, then Boston for a third time the following April as a victory lap.

After running the fastest marathons of my life in Boston, I realized that going faster on that course was not possible. The roads were too narrow, the runners were too crammed, and the hills in the late miles were too long. I also realized that I never enjoyed myself or took in all the experiences the run had to offer. There were screaming Wellesley College girls who offered kisses — I moved to the other side of the road to avoid the congestion. There were towns and monuments I never saw — I was staring down at the feet of the people in front of me, trying to get around the slower runners. Each time I raced in Boston, I started much farther back in the crowd than I finished, meaning I ran by and around thousands of runners who were, essentially, in the way. I needed to race for time elsewhere and just enjoy myself in Boston.

My first run after the Maah Daah Hey was cumbersome. Perhaps my legs just needed to be worked out to get the blood flowing. The next day, I ran five miles instead of seven. Something still felt off, though. The following day I eased off the gas and ran only three miles. I considered that perhaps it was due to the virus.

I went to see my primary care physician and explained what was going on.

"I had Coxsackievirus several weeks ago and went on a bike trip even though I was sick. Ever since then, every time I run I feel terrible and my heart rate is really high."

She listened but seemed to immediately put this into one diagnostic box—a heart problem. She ran an electrocardiogram (ECG) to look for signs of heart damage or irregular rhythm. The ECG was normal. She referred me for an echocardiogram, or echo, to see if my heart was pumping properly and then to the cardiologist. I couldn't disagree with this approach.

I asked around on a triathlon website forum to see if anyone else had dealt with similar issues. It felt odd as a physician asking the lay public for answers to health questions, but I figured I'd rather be healthy than prideful and sick. Unfortunately, the responses did not help me nail down a path forward, at least not yet.

The cardiologist read my echocardiogram as having a slight decrease in how much my heart squeezed, a measurement called the ejection fraction, or EF. A normal EF is 55 percent to 70 percent. An EF of 70 percent means that the left ventricle of the heart can squeeze out 70 percent of the volume of blood that is in it each time it contracts. The left ventricle then relaxes and fills up with blood again, back to 100 percent full. My EF was between 50 percent and 55 percent, meaning it was borderline low, especially for a fit guy like me.

My cardiologist, a caring, slightly stoic woman I admired, told me this was likely a viral myocarditis—inflammation of the heart muscle due to a virus. This seemed plausible, as

Coxsackievirus is known to affect the heart in some individuals, especially adults. She recommended abstaining from exercise for three months and then doing a repeat echo. Next time, the echo would be done immediately after walking on a treadmill.

I followed her orders of no running, but I lifted weights to keep my sanity. I had no symptoms at all lifting weights. It was high time I did some weight training, so I didn't mind the shift in gears. After years of running long distances, my arms looked like those of Olive Oyl, without any real muscular definition. My cardiologist's orders meant I wouldn't be able to get out and ride and run in the mountains for the summer, but I probably needed a break.

When it came time for the follow-up echo, my cardiologist, who was there to observe, had the tech put electrodes on my chest before asking me to start walking. They followed a protocol that increased the treadmill's speed and the incline every minute or two. The goal was to get me to the point of surrender, then quickly take an echo to look for heart malfunction.

Most echo patients are older folks and tire quickly. Having heard that one of my partners lasted a particularly long time on the treadmill, I figured going as long as possible was a badge of honor. I was no stranger to pushing myself hard and was very familiar with my maximal heart rate. I was also full of pride. So I stayed on the treadmill until I was near my max heart rate of 184 beats per minute and then called it quits.

I was not prepared for what happened next.

"Lie down, quickly!" my cardiologist barked at me. I complied immediately and experienced the most dreadful feeling of asphyxia I have ever had in my life. Who knew that lying still at a maximal heart rate would feel so suffocating?

"I have to get up!" I pleaded as the tech prepped my chest with electrode gel and started gliding the echo wand over my heart to measure my EF. "I can't breathe."

The doctor told me to lay still or I'd have to do the procedure again. I reluctantly complied, curling my toes and clenching my fists.

It paid off. I soon regained my breath.

"Your heart looks great," my cardiologist said.

"Really?"

"Yup. Get out of here and go do whatever you want."

It felt like a miracle. I was so happy to hear those words. It was September, so I could easily get in shape for Boston. Given that my kids always had a school break the same Monday as the Boston Marathon and we could stay with Melissa's parents, I could make the race an annual pilgrimage for the next decade or more. I felt much the same way that

Dan Marino probably felt about going back to the Super Bowl after making it there with ease in just his second season.

I started running again almost immediately, but I still didn't feel normal. I began to have malaise and nausea after a few runs, but I ignored it and pushed on. I successfully ran a 10K race in January, but I still could not tolerate long-distance running. Whereas I was running eighty miles per week prior to Boston, I was now barely capable of running thirty miles in a week, lest I walk home on my runs, fatigued and sick. Runs more than ten miles were impossible.

Boston in April 2015 was not going to happen.

I went back to see my PCP. She suggested that my sudden change in athletic ability was just my age catching up to me, and that I needed to adjust my goals. I was incredulous. There was no magic age limit on performance. Once I crossed the line of forty-one years and ten months, my body didn't suddenly develop an off switch. Couldn't she see that this started directly after a viral illness?

Dissatisfied with her conclusion, I enlisted the help of a former colleague, Dr. Nicole Silver, a highly intelligent functional medicine physician and a decorated triathlete who repeatedly qualified for the Ironman World Championship. Functional medicine takes a systems-based approach to look at the root cause of illness and disease. Rather than just treating the symptoms or aftereffects of an illness, functional medicine spends more time and effort trying to determine the how and why.

Dr. Silver, or Kiki as her friends know her, took an incredibly thorough history, asking me about everything from my diet to my bowel function to my sex life. I let her know that I hadn't eaten any meat aside from fish in twenty-three years, and that I never suffered from constipation, but that nausea seemed to be a huge component of my post-exertional malaise, or PEM. As far as sex went, I'd been happy in a monogamous marriage for the past twelve years.

After reviewing my medical history, she decided to look at my adrenal function and my neurotransmitters, along with a slew of nutritional measurements. This required me to spit into tiny plastic tubes, collect my urine for a full twenty-four hours, and give vials of blood. The testing revealed that my vitamin D was perilously low, but my adrenal function seemed normal. Dr. Silver recommended taking several supplements, increasing how much I slept, and decreasing my stress to help get my body back on track.

I was desperate to find my former, healthy self. After more than two decades of not eating meat to avoid contributing to farmland destruction, climate warming, and poor treatment of animals, I decided to have a steak. Not being able to run was the breaking point of my convictions.

My wife, whose Italian parents and entire extended family have a social life that revolves around food, had never seen me take a single bite of meat. One evening, I had Melissa cook me a rib eye. Tears ran down her face as she watched me take the first bite. She wasn't sure why she was so emotional about it, and neither was I. I remembered a friend telling me in college that she vomited after eating meat for the first time in years. With that in the back of my mind, I cautiously ate the steak and then waited for the regurgitation to begin. It never came. My stomach, which so often caused me problems after exercising, didn't seem to mind. Unfortunately, it wasn't a life-changing event, but I kept eating meat in hopes that it would help eventually.

My change in diet did not seem to have any effect on my athletic performance. I continued lifting weights without difficulty, but running was still a crapshoot. For a couple of weeks, I would feel pretty good and would sign up for a race, only to be unable to run again for weeks and skip the race I had just paid to enter. My frustration ebbed and flowed.

In late fall of 2015, I began to feel a little better overall. So in January, I went for a long tempo run. Tempo runs are done at a faster pace to improve running fitness. This particular run felt great from the get-go, so I picked up the speed. What a mistake. Several hours after the run, I began to feel worse than I ever had after any ride, run, or workout. For the next two weeks, I felt constantly sick. If I was not eating throughout the day, I felt ill. I craved carbohydrates, one of the only types of foods that eased the nausea.

For the next month, there would be no testing the waters, only trips to the gym a couple of times a week to lift weights. Now I was scared—a year and a half into this, I was getting worse.

In February 2016, I visited my friends Rod and Adair in California. I convinced myself to go on a slow thirteen-mile run with them on Super Bowl Sunday. I finished the run and waited to feel sick. It never came. Perhaps my constant inclination to push hard had been working against me. Maybe I just needed to throttle everything back. It would be a dramatic change to my running methods, but I had no choice.

Over the next six months, I began to run much slower and incorporated long, easy-paced bike rides. My fitness improved dramatically. I was able to tolerate longer bike rides and then trail runs. I started to feel as though this illness was gone. I fell in love with trail running, which freed me from the idea that each mile should be run at a certain speed. One mile on the trail may be uphill on technical terrain, and another may be downhill on a smooth packed-dirt single track. So I pushed when my body felt good and took it easy when my body felt tired. Soon enough, I found myself on two-hour and three-hour trail runs. I looked back at my running career and wondered why I had spent so many hours trying to run the fastest marathon possible when I could have been out training on the beautiful trails around the Flatirons of Boulder in the Colorado foothills.

Eventually, I was able to tolerate some higher-intensity rides. Perhaps even more exhilarating than going for a run was going for a bike ride before work. I would routinely start riding at 5:00 a.m., following a route from our house of exactly an hour uphill and fifteen minutes back down. As the summer progressed, the mornings grew darker, so I would ride in the pitch black with a headlight, sweating all the while. The greatest mornings were when the moon was full, and I would turn my headlight off. I would ride up the mountain, watching my shadow from the moonlight, soaking my jersey as the sun crept onto the horizon. At the top, I would be rewarded with a beautiful vista, catching the first few rays of sunlight. Even into the fall, I would ride back down while it was still dark, hitting fifty miles per hour on my narrow tires, trusting my headlight to keep me apprised of any bears, foxes, deer, or mountain lions that had wandered onto the road.

I bought the bike of my dreams during this time. With Kevin's help, I procured a Cannondale Synapse with disk brakes and electronic shifting. The bike cost me well over $6,000 with a deep discount, thanks to Kevin's business connections. I never spent money like that, but I was so happy to be active again that I said, "Fuck it," and bought it.

That fall, I decided to run my first ultramarathon, a 55K in the mountains southwest of Denver. The race's vibe resonated with me because there was no race exposition in a massive convention center, just a hand-drawn map of the parking area and the course. The runners showed up around 5:00 a.m., and the race kicked off in the dark an hour later. A stream of lights shining from the runners' headlamps lit the trail in a magical glow as we slowly ascended the first climb.

As the sun began to rise and I cruised down the first descent, I could see Denver dozens of miles off with nothing but grassland in between. The light at sunrise had a mystical quality to it. So did having a brand-new experience. I soaked it all in and felt like I was in a flow state for the next two hours. My illness was far from my mind.

As the morning progressed, the temperature rose. Thankfully, the next large climb was through a massive stand of pine trees that offered plenty of shade. Another descent brought me back to the start area, where I would snack on tater tots and bacon—a first for me in a race.

At twenty miles, I could not believe how good I felt. Not only had I just run that far, but I had done so on a technical single track up and down the mountains of Colorado. With thirteen miles to go, I started to contemplate whether I should have signed up for the fifty-miler instead. By mile twenty-two, that feeling died. The topography suddenly changed to an uphill with very little cover from the sun. I quickly ran out of water and spent the next hour wondering when I would be able to quench my thirst.

Once I reached the next aid station, I filled my bottles repeatedly, slurping down the water as quickly as I could, then asked for more. The aid station volunteer finally told me it was time to keep moving.

The next hour and a half was a long, hot, dry uphill. The arches of my feet began to ache. My body was roasting. I just needed to be done. I crested the last peak and then hobbled down the decline to the finish. More than seven and a half hours after starting, I finished my first ultramarathon, the longest run of my life, without any malaise afterward.

I must be cured, I thought.

Chapter 12

Bad Breaks

Six weeks after my ultramarathon, in late 2016, I joined CrossFit. I had been contemplating it for years, but had always been too reticent to take the leap. Because I had been forced to lift weights as an alternative to running every day over the past year and a half, I felt like I had gained enough strength to give it a go.

At first, every day at CrossFit was a challenge. It is the opposite of long slow distance. CrossFit is based on high-intensity interval training. That includes lifting moderately heavy weight at breakneck speeds. In my introductory class, I felt a sense of breathlessness and panic that I had felt only once before in my life—after lying down for my treadmill echo.

Even though I was struggling, I loved discovering new ways to challenge myself and feel fit. If the first rule of Fight Club is never talk about Fight Club, then the first rule of CrossFit is *always* talk about CrossFit. People who drink the Kool-Aid can't seem to stop proselytizing CrossFit. Elon Musk talks less to the media about electric cars and Dogecoin than the average CrossFitter tells their coworkers about their workout of the day or their fitness rebirth.

There are different prescribed weights for each workout for men and for women. Even the women's prescribed weight was far more than I was capable of. I felt most accomplished when I was able to keep up with a few of the women in my class. As for the men, unless we were running or climbing the ropes, I was just about dead last every time. Yet I loved every minute of it. My arms and legs changed shape and size. I felt strong. I could see the improvements in my workouts and the mirror.

I felt like a part of the CrossFit community at my gym. The owners were wonderful people, the coaches were sharp, and the members were welcoming and nonjudgmental, even about a skinny-armed runner joining their ranks.

As 2017 rolled along, my fitness improved in a way it never had before. I found myself gradually running faster and faster. I was even going for runs *after* the demanding CrossFit workouts. I ran the fastest mile of my life at CrossFit and a personal best at the famous BOLDERBoulder 10K. I bench-pressed more than I ever had in my life. And I was having fun.

In June, Melissa and I traveled to Barcelona to see our close friends, Jason and Barclay, who had moved there from Boulder. A trip to Spain was a perfect opportunity to see their new life and for Melissa and me to leave the country for the first time together without the kids.

From Barcelona, Melissa and I went up to Costa Brava, staying in a five-star hotel whose brunch on the terrace with a view of the Mediterranean made the start of each day a two-hour delight. I got up early each day while Melissa slept in, running along the coast while watching the sunrise. Our trip was inspiring, and Melissa and I left feeling more love for each other than we had in years.

Back home, I decided to parlay my fitness into a half-marathon in October and then a marathon in November. That October, I ran the fastest half-marathon of my life. I had a sub-three-hour marathon in my sights.

Four weeks before my November race, those old feelings of exhaustion began to reemerge. I stopped eight miles into a twenty-mile run with Kevin, who was training alongside me for the marathon. Something was off. I took some time to rest before I went for my last long training run ten days later. I ran the first twenty miles of it without any fuel, so I took energy gels the last four miles and got home feeling spent but satisfied. Four hours later, I realized there would be no marathon in November.

It was back.

The next four weeks, I felt as though I had the worst viral illness of my life around the clock. At work, for the first time in my career, I started to look around for places to sit down. I had been on my feet constantly at work for a decade, and suddenly I felt too sick to stand or concentrate.

I made it to the marathon, but not to race. I was there supporting Kevin. The night before the race I was in agony, wondering what the hell was happening to me.

Instead of this being a turning point for me, obstinate as I was, I returned to CrossFit in December, after I started feeling better. By the middle of February, I was back to running again. In late February, I slipped and fell on the ice-packed roads about four miles from my house. I knew immediately that something was wrong with my foot, so I called Melissa and had her come pick me up.

That night on the couch as I began to massage my foot, I went to straighten my knee out and heard a disturbingly loud snap. I flexed my knee again and upon straightening it, I heard the same awful sound. By morning, both my foot and my knee hurt enough for me to get them checked out. X-rays on my foot were normal, but I was diagnosed by my partner Jeff with a turf toe, a common football injury when the big toe is forcibly cocked up and tears the ligament around the toe joint.

Turf toes can range from relatively mild to career-ending injuries. For me, it took a full year before my toe felt close to normal again. My knee was a different story. It continued to lock every time it was flexed near its limit. While the MRI did not reveal an obvious torn meniscus (the cartilage around the outside of the knee that helps cushions the joint), either it existed and did not show up or the fall caused hypermobility of my meniscus. Either scenario would put me at risk for a dreaded meniscal root tear at some point, which at my age would nearly guarantee arthritis in my knee.

After spending a few weeks on the stationary bike for exercise, I slowly returned to lifting and running, with a goal to participate in the 2018 BOLDERBoulder. I would run it for a personal best, then bike back to the start line, find my son, and run it a second time with him at a leisurely pace, going through the sprinklers, high-fiving the spectators, and eating Doritos and cupcakes along the route.

A week before the BOLDERBoulder, however, the fatigue I had just before November's failed marathon mission came back. I pushed hard on race day and finished far below my expected time. I gutted out a second lap with Owen, feeling well enough to have a beer at the finish line. Three days later, I felt sick so suddenly after a workout that I quit CrossFit altogether. I went back to long, slow, low-intensity running and biking, ignoring the nagging on-again, off-again malaise.

In September, on a steep trail run to the top of Bear Peak, I felt more energized than I had since that half-marathon a year prior. On the way down, I rolled my ankle violently, which instantly made my knee buckle. Luckily, I kept from falling and continued running. No more than five minutes later, though, I rolled my ankle again and heard a loud snap.

The fifth metatarsal is the long, narrow bone on the outside of your foot that connects to your smallest toe. A fifth metatarsal fracture is one of the most common injuries I see in our fracture clinic at work, and I knew that was what had happened to me. Thankfully, it was not very painful in the moment. I knew, however, that the pain would come soon. Again, I called Melissa to come get me and hobbled out to the road where she would pick me up.

After wearing a walking boot for a few weeks, I started using a stationary bike at home and took up swimming again—the first time since 2013. Both seemed to agree with me, and I was feeling fine afterward for the most part.

One Saturday morning, I did an interval workout on my bike in the basement and then headed to a friend's house to help her sister with a medical issue. On my way over, I started feeling so sick that I could barely keep from shaking.

That was it. I could not take feeling sick anymore. I had to do something drastic.

I took the next three months off from any aerobic exercise and limited my strength training dramatically. My new routine consisted of stretching, holding an air squat for a minute or two, doing a sustained handstand against the wall, and doing one set of bench presses simply to avoid total deconditioning.

And it worked.

It was a relief not to feel so sick all the time. Thanks to the air squats, my legs felt stronger going up and down the stairs than they had in ages. It was counterintuitive. But I wasn't content to just do a ten-minute workout. I wanted to run and lift weights until I could feel my muscles swell.

Shortly after attending Super Bowl LII in Atlanta, seeing Brady and Belichick win the Lombardi Trophy for a record sixth time, I decided to return to aerobic conditioning ever so gently. For my first outing, I went for a one-mile run. My legs felt like they were filled with lead, but I felt fine afterward. A few days later, I ran two miles and cooled down with a short walk. It was too much.

"I don't feel good," I told Melissa soon after I got home.

"You feel sick again?" she asked, concerned but not as anxious as I was. She had been hearing me talk about this illness on and off for nearly five years and didn't know what to do.

"I feel terrible after a puny two-mile run at a *really* slow pace."

"Maybe you're just tired from work," she offered.

"No. Something is not right. I am so run down."

"You should go see someone about it. I'm serious."

"I have been to so many doctors," I said, the frustration and despair coming through in my tone. "No one has helped me. I keep getting the same runaround."

I was unsure of what to do. I should have returned to see my old colleague Kiki. I looked to Melissa for help. She was busy herself, in part helping a friend with a terminal illness. I felt alone.

When Owen was born and Melissa stopped working, we lived with her parents so she could stay home without it breaking us financially. As the kids grew older, she wanted to go back to work, but did not want to take a job that didn't inspire her. Her heart was in transplant surgery, but the only opportunity to be involved in transplant surgery was at the university hospital in Denver, an hour or more away.

Ultimately, Melissa began looking for other work in the nursing field. She contacted an old friend, a surgeon named

Peter, for a reference. When she went to Chicago to visit a girlfriend, she met up with Peter, who happily agreed to give her a reference. After their meeting, she told me something was off with him. She soon learned from an old colleague that Peter had a fatal motor neuron disease. Melissa was heartbroken.

Throughout 2018 and 2019, Melissa would travel to Chicago to see Peter several times, at first socially. They would meet out at a bar or restaurant, and Peter would try to act normal, failing to acknowledge that he was dying or that anything was wrong at all. Melissa would text me or come home and say, "It's just so sad." Eventually he was walking with a cane. Then he began slurring his speech. Her visits to see Peter transformed into helping take care of him, first at his bedside in the hospital and then at his home.

I was the shoulder for Melissa to cry on. I put aside the angst and pain I was having with my own health as best I could to help her deal with the impending death of a man she considered a close friend. As my health grew more concerning, however, I needed Melissa to be there for me. She felt she needed to be in Chicago for Peter. I recognized the uncanny similarity between Melissa's care for Peter and my old girlfriend Fiona's care for her ex-boyfriend after his head injury. I felt guilty about questioning their relationship at times and confused at others. Mostly, I felt sick.

IN MY NEW POSITION AS CHIEF AT WORK, I WAS HELPING guide my department through a tumultuous corporate transformation. As part of that sea change, I was also driving to Denver to work twelve-hour days in the operating room — on top of taking care of the kids when Melissa was busy in Chicago or with her clinical rotations at Denver's public teaching hospital in order to reinstate her lapsed nursing license. I would leave the house before 6:00 a.m. and often get home around 8:00 p.m. With my illness progressing, it was sometimes tough being positive about these long, demanding workdays around my colleagues, though I was charged with leading the department through the challenging times.

Long days in clinic were not bothering me. In fact, I felt at the top of my mental game. Instead of just seeing patients, I was constantly answering emails, text messages, and phone calls from my colleagues and bosses. My office was a revolving door of nurses, physician assistants, and other surgeons pleading their cases for changes or venting about someone else's bad behavior.

The OR days, in contrast, were radically different because of the physical toll they took on my body. I loved operating. I was making a difference in people's lives. But my health issues started affecting that, too. My muscles began to cramp, and I would have to switch hands intermittently just to get a screw in someone's bone. I also felt like I had to eat in between every case. By the end of the day, I was physically drained. The following day, I often would feel horribly fatigued. Adding to my confusion about what was going on was that some weeks were fine while others were abysmal. When I wasn't worrying in anticipation of being sick, I was ignoring my illness when I was sick. I hid all this from my colleagues but discussed my inability to run when they asked what race I was doing next.

I told those who asked that I had probably been overtraining and needed a respite or that I was just taking a break from too much racing over the years. As chief, I didn't want to show any signs of having health troubles. I also didn't know what was going on, so explaining my condition would be difficult, even risky. Would I detail things from the beginning six years ago? Would I tell them that during my spells I felt flulike and fatigued—but that I was fine seeing patients?

My health began affecting my ability to do tasks at home, too. In early 2019, I replaced all the dated '90s six-inch ceiling lights in our house with smaller, modern LED lights. Just climbing a ladder or moving around the tight spaces in the attic to get to the electrical wiring was exhausting. How was I going to go on like this?

Two weeks after I finished the lighting project, I walked my daughter Reese to the bus stop as I often did on my days off.

She forgot her trumpet, so I quickly ran one block back to the house to get it. Immediately, I felt like I had been kicked in the testicles. It took days to recover.

After that, I limited how much I did at home so I could go to work with energy. I gave up tackling projects, exercising, and doing yardwork, instead running errands to stay active and relieve my boredom. I became angry when I realized my life had become what my father's had been before his death — going to Walmart several times a day and collecting screwdrivers and chairs from garage sales simply because they were cheap. He had no real hobbies and seemingly no meaningful purpose in life. He became physically and mentally frail. I hated every second of feeling feeble like he had been.

I had to find answers. So I went to see a new primary care provider who I knew was an avid cyclist. When I explained my symptoms to him, he would not listen. He asked me to go to the Boulder Center for Sports Medicine to have someone help me figure out how to train properly. I tried to tell him that my problem was that I couldn't train at all, so training properly wasn't even an option. That explanation wasn't getting me anywhere with him, so I relented and went to see if the center had expertise in overtraining syndrome, a condition athletes encounter when they ignore what their body is telling them and fail to adequately rest from training. I knew I was guilty of that. Sure enough, the ultrasound of my muscles at the center confirmed this. But the doctors there offered no solution for my symptoms.

So I decided to see an endocrinologist about overtraining syndrome. He simply shrugged and asked me why I was in his office, and then told me to gain some weight. I sought a second opinion from another endocrinologist, who said he had never heard of overtraining syndrome. But after doing some research, he agreed that it was a likely explanation for my health condition.

My health continued to worsen over the next six months, and I wondered if I had a neurological disease. So I saw a neurologist to address my muscular fatigue and cramping. She specialized in multiple sclerosis as well as diseases of the brain, spinal cord, and peripheral nervous system. She was tall, fit, and attractive, about my age, and married to a triathlete. She was smart and seemed to understand the magnitude of my problem. She started with a very thorough assessment.

"What symptoms are you having?" she inquired.

"When I am in the operating room, my forearms sometimes spasm and cramp during repetitive stuff, like putting in screws to fix a fracture. At home, my jaw muscles tire out, and I have to stop chewing in the middle of eating a bite of pizza. It's crazy," I said. "This all started after a viral illness."

"When was that?" she asked, looking up from typing her notes.

"2014."

"You've been dealing with this for a really long time," she said, the concern coming through in her tone.

"Yeah. It's been a long road," I said. "I thought I was all better for about eighteen months at one point, but then I got sick again. Since then, I have been bouncing around from doctor to doctor trying to find answers, but frankly, no one is taking me seriously."

"Do you ever have numbness or pain in your chest?" she asked. "Or feel like you have a tight band around your chest?"

"No. I did have some numbness in one leg that lasted a couple of months and then the other. That's gone now. I have been getting that for years when I do shoulder replacement surgery. I lean up against the operating room table with my hip while I operate to get the best angle of approach. That always goes away shortly after the case. But then it didn't go away for a while. I also had numbness on one side of my genitals and groin for a couple of weeks, but I chalked that up to my lumbar spine."

After hearing all my specifics, the doctor considered that I might have transverse myelitis, an inflammatory condition of the spinal cord that can be triggered by a virus. I wasn't convinced, however, because not all my symptoms matched the ones I knew about the disease.

I started to wonder if this was myasthenia gravis, a condition in which the immune system attacks the communication between nerves and muscles. The more a person with myasthenia gravis does, the weaker they become, so they need rest to help restore their strength. This diagnosis was a stretch, though, since those with the condition don't typically feel ill after exercising like I did.

I also wondered if I had multiple sclerosis given my episodes of numbness, but based on my other symptoms, my neurologist ruled it out.

I had read about ME and considered this briefly, too, but from what I read, I definitely did not meet the strict diagnostic criteria.

When the MRI of my cervical and thoracic spine turned out normal, my neurologist wasn't sure what to make of my condition. I was no closer to finding an answer.

IN JUNE 2019, I TRAVELED TO FRANCE FOR A CONFERENCE on shoulder surgery. I had planned the trip a year in advance but had been anticipating it for a decade, so canceling because of my health was out of the question. Even though I didn't feel well and got only temporary relief after eating—which, as usual, I felt the need to do constantly—I was at least able to walk around.

I returned to work for several weeks and felt better than I had most of the spring. That July, Melissa, the kids, and I took a trip with friends to Greece, which I tolerated better than France. Although I had a setback—I got sick immediately after putting Reese on my shoulders for a picture—my sickness waned, and my energy increased as the trip went on.

In the weeks after our trip, I returned to some light strength training. In August, when both Owen and Reese were in middle school together, I started riding my bike the mile to school with them when I was off work. By September, this trip and my "workouts" were becoming intolerable.

Professionally, I was having a capital year. In addition to navigating all the changes at work, I was chosen to be a regional chief and received several recognitions for my accomplishments. The work was demanding, though, so in the fall, I took two weeks off to rest and complete a four-day meditation course, with the idea that perhaps some of my illness might be related to the stresses of work and life. It was physically difficult sitting on the floor all day, but eventually, I was able to do it without feeling sick. Although meditating proved helpful psychologically, ultimately, my leave did little to improve my overall physical health.

By this point, my health began to complicate other areas of life I had taken for granted. Some evenings halfway through a bottle of beer, I would suddenly feel sick the way I did after overexerting. Lifting heavy objects or weights made me nauseated. Worse yet, sex led to the same thing. I searched the medical literature and surmised my autonomic nervous system was playing a part in all of this. Some literature implicated it might be my cells' inability to produce energy, too. I remained perplexed. I wanted answers.

Little did I know they were about to come to me from an unexpected source.

Scott Simpson was an acquaintance from the triathlon forum I'd been keeping up with for the past five years. Scott had been racing Ironman triathlons when he developed ME. His symptoms totally abated a couple of times before he fell prey to unremitting illness that would keep him from exercising or living a normal life. His symptoms were so severe it was hard to consider that we might have the same illness. He reached out to me that fall to see how I was doing. I replied that I was not making the progress I wanted. In December, I started to get even worse and told him such. He responded to me, describing his own battle and advising me about mine:

My health goes up and down each day—often periods of nausea—but what has been disturbing is that I've had four episodes of waking in the middle of the night (like 2 am) to vomit and simultaneously defecate. I don't eat after 6 pm, and it's not food poisoning or the flu. It is a qualitatively different feeling and experience from those.

I've also had two episodes where my blood pressure plummets and then it is hard to breathe, and I'm quite sick for four or five days after. I did have these episodes a few years ago, but not for two years—coincidentally when I started rapamycin.

I was an idiot in January and thought I could push some snow off the sidewalk. Took about six weeks to get back to being able to walk for thirty minutes on flat ground, slowly, not carrying anything. My routine is to walk fifteen minutes to the dog park, sit around while she plays, walk home. But I am having a rough week, so driving the two to three minutes.

I had two early remissions from mild ME when I got back into full-on triathlon training and racing, but I've been sick now since December 26, 2014. That was the last day I was able to ride my bike.

I am healthier than almost every other person with ME I know . . . and I know a lot.

Michael, your objective has to be to avoid an "attack" at all costs, for you will only make yourself sicker, as you've noted. You have to suck it up and change your behavior to avoid your attacks. Reward yourself for not bringing on attack symptoms.

Michael, I'll say it again because the quality of your life depends on it: trying to maintain minimal fitness is the least of your priorities. You must stop exercising and find out where your exertion limit is, and then stay the f*ck below it.

I considered whether Scott was right. Perhaps I would wind up like him. The thought nauseated me. He had gone from Ironman to being unable to shovel a sidewalk. Could I, too, have ME?

Chapter 13

Surgeon, Interrupted

In early January 2020 as my illness was progressing, I heard the tragic news that Rodney, the brother of Ryan, our friend and companion in Europe who passed from a brain tumor, died. He was skiing with his adult sons at our local ski mountain in late December and was found down on the ground on one of the runs after an unwitnessed crash. He died on January 1. I was dumbstruck. In the years since Ryan's death, his mother had developed dementia and died. Now his brother was gone, too. His father, suffering from Parkinson's disease but still going strong, had now lost his only remaining child and immediate family member.

Rodney's funeral service, the largest I have ever attended, would be the last time for over a year that I would go to a public gathering of more than a dozen people.

As the pandemic hit full force in the States, I was wondering if I, too, was going to die from my illness. I thought about Rodney's funeral and the hundreds of thousands of people across the United States and far more across the globe who would die of COVID-19—alone in the hospital, unable to hold the hands of their loved ones. Further, their friends and family would be unable to gather to comfort each other, pay their respects, or celebrate the lives that were now over.

Selfishly, I wondered if I would simply be forgotten if my illness or COVID-19 took my life. Forgotten because there would be no memorial service and forgotten because I had been mostly housebound and out of touch with my coworkers and social circle as a result.

These thoughts about death that swirled around my brain would come to be painfully real concerns for a dear friend of Melissa's and one of mine.

IN 2020, THE SMALL GAINS IN HEALTH I'D MADE IN THE fall of 2019 vanished. Even without a long day in the operating room, I would feel nauseated, like I had the flu. So after five years, I returned to see Kiki Silver, my functional medicine doctor. I told her I thought I was battling overtraining syndrome and that it was getting worse without even exercising. She examined me as I described how my heart rate had been noticeably high simply doing surgery over the past few months and now even going up and down stairs. Somewhere in the back of my mind was the diagnosis of ME, but I still hoped it was something less nebulous, a disease with a definitive diagnostic test and a known treatment.

At the end of the appointment, Kiki and I sat across her desk from each other. She looked worried. I thought she was going to start crying. Did she think I had some progressive terminal illness? She carefully explained to me that I had dysautonomia, a problem with the autonomic nervous system where patients have poor regulation of autonomic functions, such as blood pressure and heart rate. *Thank God*, I thought. I was prepared for her to tell me something worse. She went on to compare what I had to POTS.

Postural orthostatic tachycardia syndrome, or POTS, is a common form of dysautonomia, often affecting female teenagers. It causes a rapid drop in blood pressure with standing up, dizziness, and even fainting. Kiki recommended that I treat the dysautonomia the same way that POTS is treated, with compression stockings, lots of water, and as much as three grams of salt every day. She was confident that with these modalities and a medication that raises blood pressure—midodrine—I would be able to feel better and eventually exercise again.

I took the midodrine, but noticed no improvement in my heart rate or symptoms. Additionally, I experienced some of the more common side effects, including getting goosebumps all over my body and having difficulty urinating. I also experienced an undocumented side effect that perhaps men experience and don't admit to—shrinkage. Every day on midodrine was like when George Costanza on *Seinfeld* had just gotten out of the pool. Not cool. I stopped the midodrine and things returned to normal. I had to celebrate the little victories.

I tried a few other medications Kiki recommended, including a beta-blocker to slow my heart rate. That didn't work. We also considered pyridostigmine, used to treat myasthenia gravis, but I never took it.

There are tons of theories on both overtraining syndrome and ME. These include problems with glucose transport into cells, mitochondrial dysfunction, immune system activation, neuroinflammation, low testosterone, adrenal dysfunction, gut microbiome changes, low carbohydrate intake, and more. I am a believer that the mitochondria are likely involved in the disease process of ME based in part on the lack of *battery power* I have felt in my muscles at times (truly nonscientific). If nothing else, it deserves a lot more research.

The mitochondria are known as the powerhouse of the cell. By producing an energy molecule called ATP, the mitochondria power each cell's biochemical reactions. Interestingly, the genetic code for the mitochondria is inherited exclusively from the mother and is thought to be the DNA from bacteria that were engulfed by our ancient ancestors' cells.

I tried to address some of these theories with more lifestyle changes, dietary modification, and nutritional supplements. I read *The Wahls Protocol*, a book by a physician whose multiple sclerosis improved after she adopted a paleo diet. I tried this, thinking it could apply to a broad array of illnesses, as she suggested, and got worse. I went gluten-free to no avail. I took D-ribose to aid in skeletal muscle recovery, L-carnitine, CoQ10, and nicotinamide riboside to boost my cells' energy production in the mitochondria. I didn't see any improvements, so Kiki recommended I get off all the supplements. She ordered a brain MRI, labs, and an electromyogram with nerve conduction velocity studies (EMG/NCV). The EMG/NCV uses needles inserted into arm and leg muscles to evaluate electrical activity of the muscles and nerves. It can detect ALS, myasthenia gravis, peripheral nerve injuries, muscular dystrophy, and more.

My EMG/NCV and MRI came back normal, and my labs did, too, for the most part. My bloodwork showed normal testosterone and thyroid levels, two areas I'd been concerned about, but it also revealed low levels of DHEA-S, a weak hormone that indicates adrenal gland function. Most endocrinologists consider DHEA-S unimportant, not ascribing any one illness to low levels of DHEA-S nor finding DHEA-S supplementation to treat any known disease. However, some functional medicine practitioners believe it's important. Kiki recommended I supplement my DHEA-S, but as I grew sicker, it was obvious that my issues were deeper than secondary adrenal hormone levels.

I began to track every part of my life to try to make sense of what was going on. I recorded in a notebook what I ate, how much I weighed, how many hours I slept, how many steps I took, how I felt on a scale of one to ten, and so on. I took my blood pressure and heart rate constantly. I cut tons of foods out of my diet—like chocolate, kombucha, and dairy—to see if they were affecting me. But the only thing I knew for sure was that physical activity made it worse.

By early March 2020, I was struggling to get through each day at work. I needed to eat every hour or two and still felt sick in between. As COVID-19 became a global pandemic, the stock market crashed and so did I. On March 11, I broke down and told my colleagues that I had been sick and hiding it for years, and that I had no choice but to take a leave of absence. I did two last surgeries on Friday the thirteenth, went home, and lay in bed for the next two months straight, often in tears, always in agony.

Right when I left work, the whole world went into crisis mode. As I grew sicker and sicker, I was told I simply wasn't a priority. My neurologist, who, like Kiki, was digging deep to find an answer, was made into a hospitalist and bid me adieu. I felt abandoned. I was terrified. The sicker I got, the less I was able to get help.

Late in March, my brother flew out to visit me, risking exposure to the coronavirus on the flight. What he found when he got there was worse than he'd expected. I was leaning on my side with a blanket over me, barely able to sit up on the couch and groaning while Melissa rubbed my head in disbelief. I sobbed as much from discomfort as incredulity and worry about my future.

"I'm so sorry you're going through this," Kevin said, fighting back tears as he sat down beside us. "What can I do for him?" he asked Melissa.

"Just you being here is huge," she said.

"You look better than I thought you would, dude," Kevin said in an attempt to cheer me up, just as he had during Ironman Wisconsin.

"I feel like I want to die," I squawked. "I feel like I have the flu and mono and a peptic ulcer and the worst tequila hangover of my life, all at the same time. I just don't know what's wrong with me. I have to eat, but I don't want to, because I'm so nauseated and feel so sick. But if I don't, it makes me worse for days."

Kevin had seen me feel sick before, but I'd always pushed through it, optimistic that I would beat it. "We have to figure this out," Kevin whispered. "I wish I could do something."

Weeks earlier, Kevin got his first glimpse of just how serious my condition was. While out on a short walk, I called him. Midsentence, I broke down and began to cry, telling him my condition was worsening without exercise provoking it. Worse yet, I couldn't stop it. I regained my composure and walked home after finishing our call. I went straight to the basement, sat on the bed in the guest room, and broke down again. "I don't want to be a sick person," I wailed aloud as tears ran down my cheeks. Melissa came in to investigate. She, too, was taken aback at my sudden realization that I was sicker than I had ever let on.

Before Kevin's visit, I had enough good days that it allowed me to keep going at work and do small tasks, like shop for furniture with Melissa for our newly renovated house, though I would constantly sit down at each store and often have to retreat to the car to rest or find something to eat. I had hopes that I would suddenly feel better and be able to make it out to see Post Malone in what turned out to be Denver's last major concert before the pandemic. Because I was in no shape to go anywhere and everything was rapidly shutting down, there was little choice but to stay at home.

Over the next several months, I got little relief from the television. I generally do not watch any series on TV, but I love sports. The moment I left work, though, all live sports ceased. The NBA suspended play from March 11 to July 30. Major League Baseball postponed Opening Day until late July. There was no preseason NFL. It sucked. I desperately needed a distraction. Reruns of the Mets World Series run from 1986 weren't cutting it.

We decided to watch an Adam Sandler movie to raise my spirits. *Uncut Gems* had just been released, and we assumed it would be funny. It was not and didn't try to be. In a normal emotional state, I would have needed a few drinks to relax after such an anxiety-inducing flick. In my ailing, delicate state that evening, watching that movie nearly sent me over the edge. For the first time in my life, I realized I had lost my sense of humor.

I greatly appreciated Kevin coming out to see me. I worried about him flying home and bringing COVID to his family. He didn't seem to mind the risk—or more likely, he hid his concerns from me. I am sure it was frightening to see his twin brother so sick. When I thought I might have MS, he worried about the incidence in both identical twins. His visit also must have been boring. I could barely talk. I cried. I had trouble eating. The weather was wintry. He was a trooper just for sitting there with me.

My relationship with Melissa took on new meaning. We had our ups and downs as all married couples do over the nearly seventeen years we'd been married. Once I left work and was at home sick, Melissa took incredible care of me. She sat with me. Lied down with me. Made me food whenever I needed it. She rubbed my back to ease my pain and stroked my hair. I felt closer to her than I had in years. Although I had been critical of her actions many times in the past, I was nothing but loving to her while she took care of me. I needed her — not just her caring for me, but her love for me. I felt so afraid. I needed her reassurance that no matter what, she would be there for me. It was a role reversal on many levels.

In my career, I spent endless hours taking care of others, often at their worst physically and emotionally. I saved people's lives on occasion when life-threatening infections appeared, but mostly I fixed what was broken and eased an incalculable amount of suffering. I was also the one who took care of Melissa after her knee surgeries, her C-sections, and her wrist surgery, then leading up to her Crohn's disease diagnosis and after Nonina's death. Now I needed Melissa to take care of me and to ease my suffering. If only I could find a doctor who could help do the same for me.

"I will always be here for you," Melissa assured me as I lay in bed one day shortly after I took my medical leave from work. "I love taking care of you."

"But what if I get even worse? I may not be able to do anything. Do you remember all those people in the movie we watched?" I asked, referring to a documentary about ME patients that revealed how many become socially isolated and abandoned by loved ones. I didn't think I had ME when we watched it, but it didn't matter. The images of those bedridden people in dark, quiet rooms were haunting me.

Chapter 14

Mourning Routine

In the weeks following Kevin's visit, I experienced a new set of symptoms: intolerance to stimuli. Bright lights bothered my eyes. Loud noises were painful. Walking outside into the cold made me violently ill—my body shuddered, and my abdominal muscles spasmed. As fate would have it, we had record snowfall in Boulder that year. Was this a cruel trick God was playing on me? Was I being punished for the sins of another lifetime? I pondered why such a fate would befall a person who spent his days trying to heal the sick and injured.

Not that I am a perfect person by any stretch of the imagination, but I am confident that if I stood before Saint Peter, the final analysis of my life would be that I helped my patients and strangers alike with good intentions and a firm commitment to doing what is right. I have tried to be a good son, a dependable friend, and a faithful, devoted husband and father. But that sort of thinking is not productive. I have seen firsthand in medicine the wicked shake off devastating injuries, while many kind souls suffer unfortunate fates as a result of either a bad injury or complications.

As my intolerance to lights, sounds, and temperature progressed, the flulike hangover feeling became omnipresent. I felt as sick as I could ever remember feeling from the moment I woke up until the moment I lay my head down at night. A hot shower provided no respite as it had in the past. In fact, it made things worse. Standing for a few minutes in the shower would exhaust me. My heart would pound in my chest, often at 140 beats per minute.

I had read stories of ME patients who have such limited energy that they crash for several days simply from brushing their teeth, leaving them bedridden or unable to interact with others. Activities of daily living (ADL) and personal hygiene are a luxury some ME patients can ill afford. Moments of despair set in as I imagined my condition progressing to that point. Each trip up the stairs made my legs feel like they had run out of battery power. And each trip felt like a litmus test for my future. The heavier my legs felt, the more out of energy I was, the bleaker my future looked. Even tapping the numbers on the microwave left my arm muscles weak and uncoordinated.

Perhaps the worst symptom yet, though, was the unrelenting need to sleep. Since residency, I had been incapable of sleeping more than seven hours per night. This allowed me to get a lot done, but Melissa lamented that I was rarely in bed next to her when she awoke, weekend or not. For years, my routine was to go to bed at 9:30 p.m. and get up at 4:20 a.m. Each morning, I would brush my teeth, then go make tea and my after-run breakfast—fried eggs, spinach, cheese, and Cholula on toast that went in aluminum foil, then plasticware, then an insulated lunchbox to keep it warm while I ran. Along with that, I would pack a massive glass of unfiltered apple juice to replenish the thousand calories I had just burned. I would be in the car at 4:45 a.m., running with my friends at 5:00 a.m. sharp. On Wednesdays, we ran with an official group, coached by a four-time female Olympian who, at age fifty, could still outrun all of us.

By 6:30 a.m., I was off to work, where I would shower and be ready to do surgery or see patients in clinic by 7:30 a.m. Many nights the stress of being a surgeon would keep me awake for an hour or two between two and four in the morning. Other nights I'd wake up at 3:45 a.m., lying there waiting for the alarm to sound. Now, with this illness, I found myself sleeping ten or more hours some nights. Even if I wasn't sleeping the whole time, I would often spend up to twelve hours in bed. Instead of ruminating about surgeries the next day, I lay there despairing about my flagging health.

I replaced my morning routine with a mourning routine.

Suddenly, sleep was not refreshing anymore. I now woke up feeling as exhausted as when I went to bed. This did not bode well for me. Because of my cold intolerance and my need for so much sleep, I started sleeping in the basement, where our kids would not wake me up at night as they spent the last of their boisterous, youthful energy, or in the morning as they got ready for virtual schooling. Daytime I would sit for hours on end groaning on the couch. The kids, with nowhere to go, stared at either their laptop screens for Zoom class or their father. I felt like an animal at the zoo. I couldn't escape the wondering eyes of my children as they must have been thinking, *What the hell is wrong with Dad all of a sudden?*

On my better days, I was able to muster the energy and concentration to read for a few hours. Books took my mind off my illness. Some resonated with me because of my situation, like Viktor Frankl's *Man's Search for Meaning*. I wondered how the hell anyone could keep a positive attitude under such horrible circumstances. I felt nothing redeeming about the shitstorm I found myself in. His message was not lost on me, but I felt too sick to stay optimistic.

Another inspiring book I came across was *Chasing My Cure* by David Fajgenbaum. He and I graduated from the same small high school in Raleigh, albeit years apart. In the book, Fajgenbaum goes from an insanely fit, successful college quarterback at Georgetown University to losing his mother to brain cancer to nearly dying himself of a mysterious illness while in medical school. His illness confounds his doctors and returns repeatedly, nearly delivering a deathblow each time. Fajgenbaum uses his brilliance and clinical acumen to help diagnose himself, urging his doctors to perform a lymph node biopsy that would prove he had a rare, often fatal, malady called Castleman disease. Even with a diagnosis in hand, repeatedly his life is threatened by the disease due to the lack of effective treatment. Each time the disease returns, he is hospitalized and on the brink of death as his doctors pump his weakened body full of medicines so toxic that they nearly take his life. Fajgenbaum delves deeper and deeper into researching his disease, uncovering treatments from far and wide, until finding one that works for him. He then decides to focus his entire career on helping others with the disease. The book motivated me to summon the strength to press on, looking for a way to get better.

There were days I felt so sick that I contemplated whether I had COVID on top of whatever progressive illness had been plaguing me for years. One night, while alone in the basement with the space heater blasting, I felt so sick I began to wonder if I was going to die. I contemplated whether I would ever see the sunrise again. Knowing how sick I'd been without COVID, I worried I would not survive getting it. My autonomic nervous system was short-circuiting on its own and surely would not fare well with a viral illness known to cause a massive inflammatory response. So instead of waking up Melissa and having her take me to the emergency department, where COVID loomed and where absolutely nothing might be done for me, I took my chances at home.

Over the next couple of weeks, my energy waxed and waned. There were many days that a twenty-minute phone call with someone from work would put me back in bed for the rest of the day and result in a crash for a couple more days. Helping myself at that point felt nearly impossible. How did Fajgenbaum do it? I searched health-related websites for answers, including Phoenix Rising, which is dedicated to ME. Its message boards are filled with personal testimonials that range from inspiring to shocking and depressing. Benjamin Moore has fewer paint colors than ME has unique stories. Case in point, one person with ME found out that a GI infection was causing their symptoms and was helped with antibiotics. Another got sick from antibiotics. Some got better with thyroid treatment. Others found relief after starting treatments aimed at pancreatic insufficiency. Why wasn't there one unifying cause or treatment? Which path would I go down? Was my illness even ME? The unrefreshing sleep I was now experiencing seemed to suggest so.

The medical literature offered me little insight into treating dysautonomia or ME. Review articles existed, but very few clinical trials were published. Treatments were often vague or too numerous to be helpful. The cause of ME was not clear, nor was the mechanism of disease—that is, the cellular and molecular problems that trigger it.

I awoke one morning in early April, still feeling all the effects of my illness, but with a new symptom: terrible tooth pain. I was loath to believe I could be having another problem in my life. The tooth had a crown placed on it years before and never had felt right. Food would get trapped behind it every time I ate. Eventually, my dentist placed a new crown, which felt much better at first. Over time, however, the same issues arose. I had no pain, just trapped food, so I ignored it, not wanting any further dental work. Suddenly, though, the tooth ached. I was unable to bear chewing on that side of my mouth. Hot and cold liquids and food bothered it immensely.

I was in too much agony from my other symptoms to do anything about it. So I put up with it as long as I could, chewing my food on the right side of my mouth. When the pain became a problem all day instead of just the mornings, like it first did, I emailed my dentist. He quickly replied, telling me he worried that I might have a crack in the root of the tooth. He suggested I seen an endodontist. I might need a 3D CT scan of the tooth and possibly a tooth extraction.

But when I contacted the endodontist he referred me to, I was met with the stark reality that COVID meant endodontists were seeing patients for emergencies only, such as abscesses. I did not fall into that category. So I kept ignoring it. I had bigger problems to handle. And soon, I would have much greater suffering to deal with.

Chapter 15

Thor's Hammer

Early one April day, when I had enough energy to sit on the front porch in the sun for an hour or two, I got a call from one of the physician leaders at work. Jon, a surgeon who like me also had an identical twin brother, had been a mentor throughout my leadership journey. I also considered him a friend. He was calling to check in on me, as he did from time to time. When I told him I couldn't see my neurologist because of the pandemic, he assured me that he would help me find a new neurologist and made a few phone calls.

A few days later, I had a phone visit with a new neurologist who was willing to entertain the idea of dysautonomia as the root cause of my problems. She told me about a treatment known to help some patients, an infusion of immunoglobulin called IVIG, a blood product consisting of antibodies pooled from hundreds of donors. Antibodies are the part of the immune system that fights off foreign invaders, including bacteria and viruses. The neurologist explained that IVIG had been successfully used to treat certain autoimmune nerve disorders, such as Guillain-Barre, a condition where patients suddenly become paralyzed after a viral illness. She also cautioned me about its possible side effects, including making the blood more viscous, which could lead to headaches, blood clots, or even stroke. I understood the risks and said, "Let's do it." If there was even a 1 percent chance the IVIG would get me out of the hell I was in, it was worth it to me.

A couple of weeks later, I was in a chair in my medical office building's infusion center, just down the hallway from the department of orthopedics, where I had been seeing patients and presiding as chief a month before. To prepare for the IVIG infusion, I got IV fluids to hydrate me so my vascular system was ready to accept the viscous fluid and Benadryl to decrease the likelihood of allergic reaction or side effects.

During my six hours in the chair, several colleagues from other departments passed by, giving me quizzical and sympathetic looks. I'm sure they were wondering why I was hooked up to an IV alongside their own patients, but not one of them dared to ask me why I was there.

After the first infusion, I had a slight headache but nothing worth mentioning the next day when I returned for my second round. As far as I was concerned, the first infusion was easy. Sitting up in a bright room with lots of beeping for six hours was the challenging part. The nurse again gave me IV fluids but held off on the Benadryl because it made me groggy the day before. When the infusion was over, I headed home and rested for the remainder of the day.

No more than three hours after going to sleep that night, I awoke abruptly feeling like Thor's hammer had just made solid contact with the top of my skull. Any slight movement made the agonizing pain in my head skyrocket. Unable to stand the throbbing, I crawled out of bed and up to the first floor. I was dizzy. My heart was pounding. Was I having a stroke?

I rested there for a few minutes, then went upstairs to wake up Melissa.

"I think I might be dying. Something is really wrong," I said before turning quickly around and heading back down to the living room to lie on the couch. Melissa was startled. She jumped out of bed, came downstairs, and took my blood pressure and heart rate.

"These are really high, 178 over 115 and 132 beats a minute."

Diastolic blood pressure that elevated was dangerous. Perhaps I *was* having a stroke. She took my blood pressure again. It didn't budge. I considered calling an ambulance but did not want to risk exposure to COVID, so I asked Melissa to get me Advil and Tylenol. Then I told her to get me my phone and dim the lights—she could go lie down upstairs with her phone in case I needed her. I prayed to God or any other higher being out there for the pain to go away. After twenty minutes or so, my heart rate came down closer to 100, and my blood pressure started to normalize. I nodded off a couple of times but repeatedly awoke in torment.

By morning, the pain was somewhat better but still too much for me to move. Melissa called the neurologist's office and explained the situation. Eventually, the neurologist ordered steroids to treat what she thought was aseptic meningitis, inflammation of the membranes around the brain and spinal cord. Unlike septic meningitis, which is caused by bacteria such as *Strep* and can be fatal, aseptic meningitis is more likely to be caused by viruses, medications, or systemic inflammation and is less commonly life-threatening.

Over the next few days, the steroids helped alleviate the pain, but my headache persisted for more than a month. Each time I bent over, the throbbing would return. Shaking my head to get the water out of my hair at the end of a shower was met with instant regret.

As spring unfolded, warm, sunny days punctuated the plethora of snowstorms, leaving me alternating between shivering indoors and sitting on our front porch in shorts and a sweatshirt. Our neighbors soon realized that my car was in the driveway every day and I was often out front reading. Some asked how I was doing. Many gave looks akin to those from my colleagues in the infusion center. On the snowy days, I tried to muster the energy to help Owen build a 2,573-piece Lego Land Rover Defender or draw cute little cartoons of pigs and other animals with Reese. Many days, I struggled to stay engaged doing these activities with the kids. Nevertheless, by late April, we had a finished Land Rover and a treasure trove of illustrated pigs. I had tan legs and a bevy of used books.

Over the course of the year, I had gone from having crashes going to work to having them going to the grocery store to having them standing at the sink doing the dishes. Having a crash was like losing control in the car on an icy road. When I began to feel sick, I would start to white-knuckle the steering wheel, hoping to prevent the wreck but knowing it couldn't be stopped. I would dread what was about to happen, how bad it would get. I could feel it progressing. I would try to eat and rest to minimize the damage, always to no avail.

In May, I tried to walk for fifteen minutes to maintain some conditioning. That made me feel sick. So I tried ten minutes, then five minutes, then gave up altogether. I started to get cabin fever, so I had a wheelchair delivered to the house during the last snowstorm of the spring. Melissa could use it to take me to appointments, to the store, or just to get out of the house. The kids would wheel me around the neighborhood, racing downhill screaming and laughing. On good days, I would do wheelchair wheelies in the house. It felt good on my back, but Melissa warned me to conserve my energy.

Several weeks after my IVIG infusion and the aseptic meningitis, I realized I didn't feel constantly sick every day. I wasn't sure if this was a result of the IVIG, all the rest I had been forced to take, or the relapsing and remitting nature of my illness. Most days were still very tough, but for a few hours here and there, I didn't feel desperately ill. I tried to enjoy every minute I could.

Still, each hour of the day felt like an eternity. I considered what other hobbies or activities I could get involved in, like photography. Now that I had time for it, though, I was physically unable to take the kind of nature photographs I was interested in.

I thought about taking painting classes but decided against it, assuming it would exacerbate the fatigue and cramping in my forearm muscles. Not to mention that COVID prevented any such in-person activities. Painting classes via Zoom seemed less enticing. Eventually, I settled on learning Spanish online. I had tried to learn the language before and gotten only so far. Unlike many others suffering from dysautonomia or ME, I didn't have significant brain fog, so reading and learning a language was still possible—at least when I had the energy.

Chapter 16

Welcome to the Mansion

While I was sitting on the front porch one afternoon in May, Melissa came out front. She said she had just been on the phone. Apparently, Kristi had told her daughters that Melissa was keeping her from coming out to see me. Melissa was furious.

"Let me find out what Kristi said," I offered.

"You don't believe me?" Melissa said, nearly spitting the words out. I had seen that look of contempt from her before.

I was sick and in no mood to deal with such things. "It's not that I don't believe you, but it's hard to know what Kristi said until I talk to her."

"Fine. Believe your sister and not me. She can come out and take care of you for all I care," Melissa screamed—so loudly that some of our neighbors took notice.

I sat there in disbelief as she stormed back inside. I was incapable of caring for myself, and my wife was screaming at me for something my sister said.

The genesis of this argument had come from Kevin and Kelly's plan to visit me. When Melissa and I discussed it, I suggested that Kristi stay home because of her erratic conduct and her drug and alcohol use. I was too sick to deal with wild behavior or the tension between Melissa and Kristi, who didn't get along very well.

Kristi felt hurt that she was not invited to come out. So she told her daughters that Melissa was to blame. Eventually, I told Kevin and Kelly not to visit. For Melissa and me, this was the worst fight of our marriage. We were both to blame.

Despite barely being able to get through each day, I decided to pack a bag and drive to Louisville to see Kevin myself. I would stop overnight in St. Louis to stay with his in-laws, the Langenbergs. Kevin would meet us there that night, drop off his rented car the next morning, and drive back to Louisville with me. As fortune would have it, the day I left, I felt reasonably good. Because of COVID, there was nary a car on the highway, so I set the cruise control and lane assist and got to St. Louis quickly. I left my house petrified that I would have to perform some necessary physical activity, such as changing a tire or walking to get help if my car broke down. Luckily, my car ran smoothly. The farthest I had to walk was to the bathroom at a gas station.

When I pulled into the Langenbergs' driveway, Mr. Langenberg came out to greet me.

"Kevin! How are you?" he asked.

Did he just call me Kevin? Surely he knows I am not his son-in-law.

"When is Michael going to be here?" he said.

"Hi, Mr. Langenberg. I am Michael. Kevin said he will be here in just a minute," I said, not knowing how else to inform him about his confusion.

The Langenbergs saw Kevin all the time. I was shocked that Mr. Langenberg mistook me for him. Maybe he'd had a long day. To his credit, as Kevin and I had gotten older, we looked more and more alike. We dressed similarly, too.

"I don't understand," Harry said.

"I am Michael. Kevin will be here in a few minutes," I repeated.

"Oh my goodness! I thought I was talking to Kevin," he said.

Minutes later, Mrs. Langenberg came out. She gave me a big hug despite the COVID warnings.

"When is Michael getting here?" she asked.

Is this really happening? I thought.

"This is Michael," Harry told her.

"What?" she asked, looking confused.

Thankfully, at that moment Kevin pulled in the driveway, and the misunderstanding came to a halt.

The next morning after he dropped off the rental car, Kevin and I headed to Louisville. Kevin drove the final leg of my journey, giving me a rest. After we got there, I enjoyed a day with Kevin's wife, Grace, and my nephews, Penn and Reed. Our sister Kelly drove from her home in Richmond that night to see me. Penn and Reed were attempting to finish the school year virtually, a challenge at their young ages. Two days into my stay, Grace took the boys to her sister's house in Atlanta for the week. Then Kevin went back to work.

Thanks to the rainy weather, Kelly was stuck inside with me, unsure how to help. I was feeling the aftereffects of my drive and had little energy to spare, so I spent a lot of time in the bedroom. When I felt energized enough to come out, we sat on the couch and talked or watched movies. I groaned and cried on the days when I felt really sick. She comforted me and told me she hated to see me like this, but that everything was going to be okay. I wasn't sure that was true.

Kelly drove me to Richmond later in the week so I could see our mother, whose memory was beginning to fail and who was looking frailer as the years went by. We drove through endless rain up and down the hills of West Virginia and into Virginia, laughing at Howard Stern on the radio for several hours. Perhaps my sense of humor was not gone for good.

When we got to my mother's house, I gave her a long hug, as I always do. She felt skinnier. She had lost muscle. I had, too.

We have always had a close relationship. Whenever I called my mother, my goal was to make her laugh. Sometimes I was so successful she cackled hysterically. I would mostly tell her stories of my life and occasionally the outrageous accounts of my friends' lives, Vincent, Luke, and Liam, in particular.

More recently, since my father died, she had less and less to tell me about her own life. Her social interactions were diminishing. We mainly chatted about the last time she had seen Kristi or Kelly. I would tell her about my health and what the kids were up to. She had eleven grandchildren and wasn't close to my kids, in part because of geographical distance and in part from her lack of effort—which I have regretted but can't change.

For the next several days, my mom and I enjoyed each other's company, having coffee together in the morning and talking as little or as much as we felt compelled to. She would make me breakfast, which was comforting even at age forty-seven. I was helpless to address what needed fixing around the house, like a broken cabinet door or a piece of furniture that required moving. She didn't care about that. She was just happy I was alive and visiting her. She felt my pain, and like Kelly, reassured me that everything was going to be okay someday.

Kristi came up with my nieces after a couple of days, and I confronted her about what she had said about Melissa. It was an uncomfortable situation, and I didn't feel like I got a genuine apology. But I walked away from it thankful that she knew her behavior was making my life even harder. Kristi did apologize to Melissa over text message after Melissa confronted her about what had happened, which helped mend things between them.

Kevin came to Richmond with the boys the night they got back from Atlanta to see our mom and drive me back to Louisville. The return drive was divine. We had all the windows down, and warm, humid air washed over us. Kevin said it was the first time he'd ever driven through the mountains of West Virginia without it raining. We stopped on the side of the road for Penn and Reed to pee a few times. Reed asked for something to eat every few minutes. We played the Grateful Dead loudly, my noise and light sensitivities having improved significantly. Nine hours in the passenger seat of his SUV seemed to fly by—a stark contrast from just a few months ago, when every hour seemed an eternity.

Back in Louisville, I stayed a couple more days until I was ready to go home to Melissa. We had spoken very little while I was gone because of our argument. In need of some independence, I took a quick trip to Trader Joe's by myself to get food for the drive home.

The next day, Kevin, the boys, and I went back to St. Louis. Mrs. Langenberg mistook me for Kevin once again. Kevin and I both laughed. The boys spent the day in their grandparents' pool, and I relaxed in a chair nearby, enjoying the fun they were having and talking to Grace's sister. Later that afternoon, I began to feel sick from my grocery trip and lay down. I missed dinner and got up before sunrise. Kevin heard me up and came out to see me off. I bid him farewell and said he should pretend to be me and say goodbye to his in-laws when they awoke. He laughed.

I left for home glad to have seen Kevin but reminded of how sick I really was. When Kevin and I used to run together, I was sharing something I loved immensely with him.

In 2016 and 2017, when I still had enough energy for exercising, we ran together in Louisville on the weekend of the Kentucky Derby. The first year I attended the Derby, Kevin's bosses, brothers who started the company Kevin was president of and old friends of ours, spoiled us with tickets to the race. They didn't just buy us any tickets, though. They bought us tickets to The Mansion, perhaps the most coveted tickets in all sports, hovering around $10,000 each.

We got dressed up for the Kentucky Oaks race on Friday, a day known for business interactions and glad-handing. It was nicer than any sporting event I had been to and popular among celebrities of all sorts, particularly athletes. At one point that day when Kevin and I got on the elevator up to The Mansion—the top-floor VIP area of Churchill Downs— I turned to him and whispered, "That is Brandt Snedeker. He's one of the top golfers in the world." The entire weekend I spotted one famous person after another, pointing them out like a bird-watcher to Kevin.

On Saturday, Kevin, Grace, her sister, and I entered Churchill Downs through the main entrance, presenting the tickets and passing through the turnstiles surrounded by thousands of people outfitted in sartorial splendor. Once inside, Kevin took us around a corner to an elevator, where an usher put bracelets on our wrists. We rode up to the top floor and were greeted in the foyer by a group of staff.

"Welcome to The Mansion," they said, as if we had just arrived at Willy Wonka's Chocolate Factory. We checked in at the desk, where we were introduced to our personal butler for the day. This pleasant young man would be able to get us anything we needed and take us anywhere we wanted. We filled out forms for commemorative handblown glass cups that would be mailed to us. Our butler then took us to our seating area, designated as a living room, which was surrounded by several other seating areas, all bordering a wide-open space without walls known as the grand area. In the central living room, rented by NBC Sports, we saw Chris Collinsworth with Tony Romo—a courting that went unrequited as Romo later famously signed with CBS Sports.

Our tickets allowed us to go down to the paddock to see the horses, stand trackside, and enter any other seating area we wished. Kevin had our butler take us down to the outdoor boxes just beyond the glass walls of the Turf Club—an area known for high-stakes betting. Standing there was Aaron Rodgers with several of his friends and NFL teammates. I was impressed.

Moving south from where Aaron Rogers' seats were, we walked toward the other end of the outdoor boxes, where Kevin had seen Tom Brady the year prior. Lo and behold, Brady was there, listening to music with his teammates, some smoking cigars, and all dressed to the nines. We stopped a few feet behind him, and I chatted with an acquaintance who was friends with Brady, looking for any reason to stay there as long as we could. For a fleeting moment, we felt like part of their crowd.

My trip to Louisville in the midst of my illness made me remember all those good times Kevin and I had together, times when I was still able to do seemingly whatever I wanted to do. Seeing Kevin again was like seeing my former healthy self. For the rest of my life, perhaps, I would have to live vicariously through him, wishing him well on his own runs, races, and adventures to places like The Mansion.

Chapter 17

You Have to Slow Down

My drive back to Colorado was rough. I felt okay for the first few hours, then started having my typical waves of nausea and malaise. My short trip to Trader Joe's was a mistake. Luckily, I had enough food to dampen my symptoms.

I made it home in time for dinner, and my family said very little as I came in the door. Perhaps they needed the break from me. After eating together, mostly in silence, I showered and went to bed. Melissa and I tried to reconnect, but the anger on both sides was still there.

I spent most of my time reading and sitting outdoors alone as the kids finished the last few weeks of remote classes. The snow had finally stopped falling in late April, and summer appeared close by.

I asked my neurologist and functional medicine doctor for referrals to two separate academic institutions. One was Stanford University, where I had found an ME clinic within the Division of Infectious Diseases. Through my internet sleuthing, I found several patients who were recommending a handful of the same places, including Stanford. I came across clinical research articles linked to Dr. Jose Montoya in the university's Division of Infectious Diseases and Dr. Ron Davis, a PhD researcher and professor of biochemistry and genetics. Their research seemed promising. The website stated that they believed in an association between viral illnesses and chronic fatigue syndrome. It also described ME as a bona fide physical ailment, not a psychological disorder. Describing ME as a psychological disorder has led to widespread disregard of the disease and blaming of patients for their symptoms. It has also led to further marginalization of those with mental illness, suggesting someone can choose to get better from the condition on their own.

I began making calls for an appointment. Stanford stated that they were currently not seeing patients in person from out of state because of COVID, so I took the soonest appointment with a physician assistant, which was several months away. Initially, I wanted to see Dr. Montoya, who, based on the research I had read, had been leading the charge in researching ME as a post-viral syndrome. I found out that Dr. Hector Bonilla had replaced him and told Melissa I wanted to see him instead. I hoped he would share the same drive to help patients as Dr. Montoya.

Among Melissa's many areas of expertise—including concertgoing and returning items she purchased months or years ago—is getting in touch with doctors for family and friends. So she began to make calls and send emails to find a way to get me into Stanford sooner. A sister of a close friend had a connection she was able to leverage to get me on Dr. Bonilla's radar. Despite being in the Division of Infectious Diseases in the midst of a historic pandemic, he reached out to me on a Saturday.

"Michael?" he said, "this is Hector Bonilla from Stanford."

"Dr. Bonilla, hi," I said, still shocked to hear from him. "Thank you so much for calling me."

"Please, call me Hector," he said in a smooth Colombian accent.

I thought this was going to be a quick conversation about my needs. Instead, it turned into an hour-and-a-half phone consultation. Fortunately, Melissa was there, and we spoke to him together on speakerphone.

"When did you first get sick, Michael?" he asked.

"I had a virus in 2014," I told him.

"Tell me about that."

I proceeded to detail my mountain bike trip to the Badlands, the workup I had afterward, and my current signs and symptoms. I told him about my athletic past, my career, my marriage, and my children. He wanted every detail. We finished with Dr. Bonilla documenting the self-reported severity of my symptoms.

"Over the past thirty days, what would you rate your fatigue level at its worst, 0 to 10?"

"Nine," I said.

"Over the past thirty days, what would you rate your fatigue level at its best, 0 to 10?"

"Four."

"Do you have more days at 4 or more days at 9?" he queried.

"Nine," I told him.

He continued asking me to characterize how refreshed I was when I woke up in the morning, how much pain I had, and how much brain fog I experienced.

At the end of our conversation, he said, "You definitely have ME."

It was the first time anyone had said that with certainty. It was a relief to have a diagnosis yet devastating at the same time.

He went on to explain his recommended treatment for patients with ME—pacing.

"You have to slow down, Michael. The more you do, the higher your risk for a crash. You are a high performer, but you can't be this way anymore."

I was overwhelmed to hear someone tell me that I could not be what I already knew I was incapable of being—a high performer. I may have been an ultramarathoner and chief of orthopedics in the past, but in reality, I was no longer either of those things, and I might never be again. But at least a doctor legitimized what I was saying.

He recommended that I stop taking supplements and start taking naltrexone, a medication used to treat alcohol and opioid dependence but that had given relief to some patients with ME in low doses. I had read about it and was willing to take it. He discussed other potential options for medications but suggested that I start with naltrexone and go from there. I agreed.

In addition to Stanford, I asked for a referral to Mayo Clinic because of their expertise in dysautonomia, one of the components of ME that affected me most—namely a constantly elevated heart rate. Scott, the fellow triathlete I communicated with online, warned me of his experience with Mayo. "No, no, no," he told me. "They perpetuate medical harm." I ignored his advice to not go but approached my evaluation there with caution. My experience would prove his warning was warranted.

I spent several weeks lining up appointments and gathering medical records. It was difficult and frustrating at times, particularly during COVID when people were learning to work from home. But I was grateful that Mayo Clinic was seeing patients in person. I'd start with a neurologist since I had an official diagnosis for a neurological condition.

After years of looking for answers to my illness, my family and I packed up our car and drove for two days to Rochester, Minnesota. We settled in for the night at a cheap hotel room just two blocks away from the hospital, with Melissa and me in a double bed and the kids on a pullout sofa. When I was healthier, we enjoyed camping together in the mountains of Colorado. This was as close as we would get to camping for the foreseeable future.

The next morning, we left the kids, who were still sleeping like two teenagers, in the hotel room while Melissa pushed me in my wheelchair from the hotel to the palatial medical office building next to the hospital. Thankfully, summer had arrived in Minnesota, and the early morning trip was tolerable.

Upon entering the medical office building, our temperatures were taken by nurses at a makeshift triage station just inside the massive front doors. From there, Melissa wheeled me to the elevators that we would take up eight floors to the Department of Neurology.

We checked in at the manicured front desk area and found a spot to wait, keeping an awkward distance from the other patients. Most of them were much older than me. Many looked far sicker. I felt out of place. Melissa held my hand and remained optimistic that we would get the answers we needed there.

My name was called after a twenty-minute wait. Melissa pushed me back to the room, and we parked my wheelchair outside the door. I got up and walked into the room, feeling horribly self-conscious. To an outsider, I looked healthy. I wasn't paralyzed. I had no cast on either of my legs. Yes, I was capable of walking short distances, but not without feeling sick hours later. I felt like a phony for being in a wheelchair.

I had an invisible illness.

Once inside the examination room, the nurse asked me to have a seat and took my blood pressure and pulse. It was colder inside than it was outside, rare for Minnesota, I'm sure. We waited a few minutes anxiously until the neurologist came in.

"Hello. I am Dr. Meier," he said with a subtle German accent.

"I'm Michael. Nice to meet you. Thank you for seeing me. This is my wife, Melissa."

He acknowledged Melissa, then turned back to me. "I have looked through your history, but let's start from the beginning. Tell me what has happened."

I started from the beginning with my bike trip to the Maah Daah Hey and went from there. He took a very thorough history, asking many questions. He didn't perform a physical exam, which was a little surprising and disconcerting for a neurologist and not what I expected from Mayo. He looked through my labs and paperwork that I brought from my workup back home. I told him about my diagnosis of dysautonomia that a functional medicine doctor had made and a local neurologist had agreed with. I used the words "post-exertional malaise" several times to describe my illness since it was my most prominent and troublesome symptom.

He explained to us that he had seen a patient just like me the year before—an ambitious physician involved in running and triathlons who suddenly and inexplicably became unable to exercise. *Hallelujah*, I thought, *I have come to the right place.* Melissa then asked, "How did he do?"

"I don't know," he replied. "I never saw him again."

"You never saw him again?" Melissa asked.

"No. With these things, we rarely figure out what the real underlying cause is," he confessed.

"So, what good is it that you saw someone else just like Michael?" Melissa wondered out loud.

He had no response. He wanted me to get a slew of tests and bloodwork that I had already done back home. I asked that we not repeat the ones I already had. Instead of agreeing, he asked us to sit out in the waiting room until he could review the records I had brought with me in further detail.

An hour later, one of the neurology nurses approached us.

"Dr. Meier would like you to get these studies," she said, handing me several sheets of papers detailing the labs and studies he had ordered along with a schedule of appointments.

I glanced through them. "These are all the things he listed when we were in the office. I asked him to cancel the ones I have already had done."

"Let me check with him," she said.

She returned after several more minutes. "He said he wants all those things repeated in our system to be sure they are accurate." We agreed, perturbed but not entirely dissuaded.

From there, I was sent to have a Holter heart monitor placed, which I'd had done twice already. The woman who put the

Holter on me was pleasant, as was everyone there, but she moved so slowly that it looked like we were watching one of our kids when they take a slo-mo video on my iPhone. Melissa and I started laughing uncontrollably. It felt like it had been months since we had the urge to laugh together.

My other appointments with cardiology and internal medicine were spread out over the next three days. Additionally, I was being referred to the chronic fatigue clinic. There was no appointment available for that clinic until September.

My cardiology appointment was scheduled the day after I was to walk on a treadmill for a VO_2 max test, which measures cardiopulmonary fitness. I tried to move the cardiology appointment up sooner, but was told I needed to complete the treadmill test first. I informed the receptionist that walking on the treadmill would be very challenging for me and make me sick. I said I would rather see the cardiologist without doing that test. She conferred with the medical staff, then informed me that I had to do the treadmill test if I wanted to see the cardiologist. Period. Given that my heart rate had been such an overwhelming issue for the past several months, I desperately wanted to see the cardiologist. After weighing the pros and cons, I ultimately relented.

When my name was called, I stood up out of my wheelchair.

"Be careful, please," Melissa begged me.

"I will. I'm just going to do enough so that I can get the test done and see the cardiologist," I assured her.

"Right this way, Dr. Gallagher," the young, pleasant technician told me. She brought me back into the lab and asked me to remove my shirt. Another young woman was there to help, as well. They both donned gowns, gloves, masks, and face shields as part of their COVID protocol. For the first time in my life, I was self-conscious about the way I looked. My muscles had atrophied. I looked droopy and weak at forty-seven. This was worse than dad bod.

After I'd undressed, the young women placed ECG stickers on my chest. Each one felt icy cold as it touched my bare skin. Then they hooked me up to a face mask that would measure my respirations. I was hoping this would help me get some answers.

As the speed and incline of the treadmill increased, I walked faster and faster, listening to the beeping of the machine tracking my heart. I kept going until my heart rate was in the high 150s and then gave up. It took very little time. I hoped this would give them what they needed and get me in to see the cardiologist. The technicians stopped the treadmill and unhooked me from the monitors. I put my cotton oxford shirt back on, and they escorted me back out to the waiting area.

"Are you okay?" Melissa asked.

"I'm fine. It was easy. I got off pretty quickly."

"Is that going to be enough?" she asked.

"It should be."

"As long as you don't get sick from this," she said.

"I know," I said, feeling worried.

We returned several hours later for my next appointment, which Melissa was able to move up a day via some persuasion of the staff. I was taken back into the cardiology department, and we saw an older gentleman, probably close to seventy. He discussed my treadmill test results with me.

"Your VO$_2$ max is way down here. Twenty-two," he said.

"Wow. That's really low. When I was running marathons, it was 55," I informed him.

"You are very deconditioned."

No shit, I thought, *my kids could tell me that*.

Instead, I told him, "I know. I have been very, very sick. I can't even walk for exercise. It makes me sick to exert myself at all."

As the conversation progressed, Melissa and I realized that this man was not a cardiologist but an exercise physiologist. He told me I was simply out of shape and needed to exercise more. My wife and I could not believe what we were hearing. He recommended graded exercise therapy. Did he not hear anything I told him? The problem was that I *couldn't* exercise. If I could, I would be exercising every goddam day of my life. Additionally, I had tried a gradual return and failed miserably, repeatedly making myself more ill each time. Worse, I was getting sicker and sicker without even exercising. I knew ME patients had pathologically low VO_2 max results like mine—not from sitting around doing nothing but from abnormal physiologic processes, like mitochondrial or autonomic dysfunction. I was there to find out what the hell I could do about it.

He said nothing about the rapid heartbeat I was having from tasks as simple as showering. He didn't address the fact that I went from running ultramarathons to getting tired going up the stairs. To boot, I looked healthier than he did. It felt like having someone sitting next to me, chain-smoking and eating a double bacon cheeseburger while watching Judge Judy telling me I should just stop complaining and live a healthier lifestyle. Did they tell paraplegics to just get up and walk? Or cancer patients to just have their cells stop multiplying so rapidly? I couldn't believe the ignorance.

We left the cardiology department after I was told to exercise more and I said to Melissa, "That's it!"

"What do you mean 'that's it'?" she said.

"I'm done. This is ridiculous. They are not even listening to me. They asked me to repeat all the labs and tests I've already had. I came here for a bespoke approach to my illness. For a fresh set of eyes. All I got was the same exact workup with even less of a patient-specific, novel tactic."

I should have known. The labs and tests, in fact, had been ordered before I even got there, I realized. This shotgun approach was not custom-tailored in any way.

Melissa implored me to just get the rest of the labs and stay around for the next two days to see what else may happen. But I had had enough. I asked her to wheel me back to the department where we were laughing earlier about the leisurely placement of the Holter monitor. Once there, I asked them to take it off me. We went back to the hotel and debated our next move.

"You don't have any other options," Melissa said. "Please just see what they have to say."

I was having none of it. I was sick of being sick. Worse, I was sick of being shuffled along a conveyor belt of patients who didn't fit into a simple diagnostic box.

"Fuck this place," I barked.

Melissa called my cardiologist back home, revealing to her what had transpired with Mayo's cardiology department. She, too, recommended I get the labs. She would try to see if she could find an actual cardiologist there who would see me —one who specialized in autonomic disorders. I greatly appreciated her interest in helping me, but I chose to call it quits. I was exhausted and didn't feel like wasting any more time or money at an institution that didn't seem to care that much to treat ME patients. I had little tolerance for people who did not have my best interest in mind.

Chapter 18

Graded Exercise Therapy

ME most often starts with a virus, but it is not one disease. There are many causes. Just as a headache can be from a brain tumor, aseptic meningitis, or dehydration, ME can be from a virus, endocrine dysfunction, GI infection, and even a spine problem in the neck called craniocervical instability (CCI). Why there are so many different causes for the same cluster of symptoms is unknown. But there are two unifying symptoms: fatigue and post-exertional malaise. Most of the ME community believe the best treatment is pacing—expending a confined amount of physical, mental, or emotional energy to prevent relapses or "crashes."

Viral infection as the root cause of such an illness makes sense to most patients, doctors, and researchers. Viruses can wreak havoc on the body, especially the immune and nervous systems. CCI is much less intuitive. CCI is a problem with the ligaments where the skull attaches to the top of the neck, an area called the cervical spine. These ligaments not only allow you to move your head, but they also stabilize it, thus protecting your brainstem and spinal cord.

The brain, brainstem, and spinal cord make up the central nervous system. The peripheral nervous system, in contrast, is made up of the nerves that come out of the spinal cord. These nerves are either motor (control muscles), sensory (provide sensation), or autonomic (control blood pressure, heart rate, and other involuntary processes). People with ME are known to have problems with the autonomic nervous system. So is ME a neurological disease? The World Health Organization believes it to be. Most ME patient advocacy groups say it is. The CDC has not, however, explicitly defined it as one.

My experience has been that this seems very much like a neurological illness with other manifestations—for example, diseases of the autonomic nervous system. The autonomic nervous system is divided into the sympathetic and parasympathetic. The sympathetic nervous system controls fight or flight. If your ancestor saw a saber-toothed tiger, her sympathetic nervous system would prepare her to either fight for her life or flee. Her pupils would widen to see everything around her, her lungs would open up to take in more oxygen, her heart rate would speed up to get more blood and oxygen to the muscles. In modern times, this is what happens during stage fright while you're speaking in public. Your heart feels like it is jumping into your throat. It also happens to be the part of the nervous system responsible for orgasm in women and ejaculation in men.

The parasympathetic nervous system is known as the rest-and-digest portion. It controls your body during ordinary situations, such as stimulating salivation and digestion, slowing your heart rate, and making you urinate.

Because your brainstem is involved in the autonomic nervous system, brainstem damage can cause autonomic dysfunction, or *dysautonomia*. Namely, sweating, blood pressure, heart rate, and other automatic functions aren't regulated properly. Instead of their blood pressure dropping slightly when standing, patients like me with autonomic dysfunction do not get the normal signal from their autonomic nerves that tells their blood vessels to squeeze tightly. Instead, their blood vessels remain relaxed and dilated, which creates blood pools in their legs. Thus, their brain gets less blood and oxygen, and their heart rate spikes to keep the blood flowing in their brain. Their bodies also don't respond normally to temperature changes. For example, they may not sweat, which cools the body when its core temperature rises, so they develop heat intolerance. They can also have cold intolerance because their blood vessels don't constrict to keep their core temperature at 98.6 degrees.

Jeff Wood, a patient who battled chronic fatigue syndrome for years after a viral infection, became bedridden at home and was plagued by post-exertional malaise. He was unable to tolerate posture changes, temperature variations, physical exertion, or even light and sound. After progressing for years without relief, he began to have neck pain. He used what little energy he had to research his symptoms. Noticing that they worsened when he was upright and improved when the foot of his bed was elevated, Jeff postulated that his neck may be the issue. He also nearly passed out when he turned his head to the right. After reading about craniocervical instability and an associated condition called atlantoaxial instability (AAI), he figured that the ligaments at the top of his cervical spine were not providing adequate stability. As a result, his brainstem was being pinched each time gravity put any force on his head, such as when he was standing.

Jeff sought the care of multiple neurosurgeons regarding his hypothesis that his neck might be the root cause of his ME symptoms, including the severe dysautonomia. He was "ridiculed, scoffed at and even met with frank hostility and derision" by these doctors. No one believed him. Then his symptoms worsened, and he began to have trouble breathing. In his mind, this all added up to brainstem compression from CCI. The autonomic nervous system controlled so much of the functions that were going awry; how could it not be the root cause?

Jeff began wearing a neck brace he purchased to stabilize his cervical spine, and voilà, he could stand up easier. While the neck brace helped with some of his worst symptoms, he remained very unwell. He found common ground on Facebook with patients who have Chiari malformation—a separate issue that causes the brain to push through the bottom of the skull, putting pressure on the brainstem and spinal cord. He also found medical literature to support his hypothesis. Then, one day, he took off his neck brace and immediately became dizzy. He had trouble moving his arms and legs, too. His heart rate skyrocketed. It was more than he could bear, and his family called an ambulance. He was admitted to the hospital. What happened next illustrates why the disregard for and misunderstanding of ME patients must change.

Jeff asked his doctors if they could put him in a halo, a medieval-looking contraption that is screwed into the skull to help stabilize the top of the spine. Four screws are attached to an outrigger that then attaches to a vest. After the patient receives a local anesthetic, the doctor places the vest on them while they are lying flat (their neck injury usually doesn't allow them to sit upright safely during the procedure). Then, the surgeon gradually tightens the screws with a wrench until there is enough pressure on the skull to keep the halo in place and the spine stable. Typically, two screws are in the skin just above the eyebrows, and two are toward the back of the skull through the hair behind the tops of the ears. When it's all said and done, the patient looks like they're wearing a life jacket with an Erector Set on top that is drilled into their brain. I placed these on numerous patients with cervical spine injuries and can tell you that the process is as cringeworthy as it sounds.

Jeff's calls for a halo went unanswered. His doctors thought he was misinformed or deranged asking for it. After all, patients just don't come into the hospital asking for screws to be drilled into their skull. However, Jeff couldn't go home. His symptoms were too severe. So, he laid in a hospital bed for nearly five months, keeping the top of his bed tilted down so the weight of his head would not put pressure on his brainstem. By that point, the doctors insisted that he be evaluated by psychiatrists, who found him to be both sane and intelligent without any delusions.

Day after day he lay there without getting any help, only accusations. His fortunes changed on his 123rd day, when the head of neurosurgery came to see him. He listened to Jeff in a way that no one had before. He considered Jeff's hypothesis plausible and ordered a CT scan of his neck. Sure enough, the CT scan confirmed instability. Jeff got his halo placed. And after 143 days in the hospital, he went home.

Having been immobilized for so long, Jeff's muscles were weak. But he was able to stand up. And then walk. His heart rate stabilized. His post-exertional malaise was gone. The inevitable energy crash never came. He started living a more normal life, doing things like going out to dinner. In total, he had spent four years in bed. Four years! In bed! I went from waiting tables and drinking nightly with my goofball buddies in Boulder to being a medical doctor in four years. Eventually, he found a surgeon to fuse his skull to the top of his cervical spine. The surgeon suggested he had issues similar to patients with Ehlers-Danlos syndrome (EDS), an inherited disorder of collagen, the protein that gives ligaments their strength and structural integrity.

Jeff's surgery cured him.

There are questions about why a viral illness can trigger ME, especially in someone with EDS. Can the virus somehow alter collagen through some inflammatory or immune cascade? No one knows at this point.

Jeff posted information about his journey on Phoenix Rising, the same website I used to search patient forums looking for answers. In doing so, he caught the attention of Jennifer Brea. Jennifer was a PhD student at Harvard in 2011 when she suddenly became ill with a viral infection. Her disability quickly progressed until she was mostly bedridden. Like Jeff, she was considered mentally ill by some of the doctors who saw her. She was desperate for answers but found very few. She documented her and others' heartbreaking and horrifying struggles with ME in *Unrest*, a documentary that won a Sundance Film Festival award in 2017. Many of the people in the film are bedridden and have been ignored or even abused by the medical community. By the end of the documentary, Jennifer's illness is no better.

I watched *Unrest* several years ago as I searched for a diagnosis, convinced at that time that I did not have ME. My symptoms were too mild and didn't match the criteria—namely, I still did not have unrefreshing sleep. The people in *Unrest* were so much worse off than I was. I never considered that I could get as sick as they were. In many ways, I was wrong. My advancing symptoms over the next two years would lead me to realize I was at risk of being bedridden at any time. The fact that Jennifer was able to make a movie despite her physical condition is a testament to her drive to help others and to her intellect.

When Jennifer read Jeff's testimonial, she recognized the similarities in their stories and symptoms. She was contacted by a vascular neurosurgeon, who had noticed that some of his EDS patients began to have unusual symptoms after a viral infection. These symptoms matched those he saw Jennifer exhibit in *Unrest*. Her MRI caught his attention, as well. Like many others, she questioned whether CCI was even a possibility. Her illness started with a virus—what did that have to do with instability of her spine? Before being evaluated further, Jennifer underwent surgery for thyroid cancer that left her with drastically worse symptoms. Like Jeff, she began to have difficulty breathing when upright or turning her head one way. And she would stop breathing altogether if her head was in certain positions. When the part of the drive to breathe that comes from the brainstem is compromised, breathing stops. This condition is referred to as central apnea. On the advice of a friend, she started wearing a neck brace similar to Jeff's. While that didn't cure her symptoms, it did help. She then contacted one of the doctors who helped Jeff, and he ordered an upright MRI to prove that she had CCI.

In a seemingly barbaric intervention, Jennifer had sharp tongs attached to her head with weights that pulled traction on her skull via a pulley and rope until she felt better. I have placed these tongs on patients in the emergency department with acute trauma to the cervical spine and spinal cord caused by diving into shallow pools headfirst or getting into severe car accidents. The tongs in those cases pulled enough traction to put dislocated vertebrae back into place, taking pressure off the brainstem and spinal cord. Patients would stay in the tongs with traction until they could be taken to the operating room soon after, where their cervical spine would be stabilized with metal plates and screws. Jennifer's X-rays taken while she had the traction on proved that her neck was unstable. After her fusion surgery, her neck was stabilized. She later underwent a tethered cord surgery, as Jeff Wood had also done. Her ME is now, in her words, "in remission."

Eight years Jennifer spent ill and mostly in bed. She was made to feel that her illness and symptoms were all in her head—even by doctors. It is hard to imagine this type of disregard and accusation on top of her illness. Jennifer continues to advocate for patients with ME and is an inspiration to so many of us. She cofounded a global advocacy network called #MEAction that serves to help those diagnosed with ME and those searching for answers. #MEAction helps get proper information out about ME via social media and the organization's website. They raise awareness and fight for education, recognition, and research for people living with ME. They have launched Twitter campaigns, including #PWME and #MillionsMissing for the millions of people who are missing out on their social lives, careers, families, and more. The mantra of the #MillionsMissing is "I got a virus and never got better."

I live those words every day.

After reading about CCI, I began to wonder if it could be the cause of my symptoms. I doubted it based on my lack of neck pain and the intermittent nature of my illness, but I would be remiss if I did not find out for sure. So I read through a few journal articles and websites trying to find out more. I was surprised to see that Johns Hopkins had published an article about three patients whose ME symptoms resolved after anterior cervical discectomy and fusion (ACDF), a surgery for herniated discs and/or arthritis, performed far more commonly than surgery for CCI. I asked my friend Spiro about it. He told me he'd had patients who described weird, vague symptoms that went away after he performed the surgery. He said he never knew what to make of it.

I hoped a simple disc issue could explain my problems and started searching for an upright MRI. I found a clinic south of Denver that had been doing an increasing number of flexion-extension MRIs over the past year or two to look for CCI—likely as a result of the documented association with ME. These specific upright MRIs can create images of the spine during flexion (bending forward) and extension (bending backward), which was important to see if the position of my neck was causing my symptoms. I contacted them and set up an appointment to have one done.

The day of the MRI I was feeling dreadful. I drove down to the facility and sat in my car in the parking lot to call the phone number given to me. A woman wearing gloves and a mask came out with a clipboard. I opened my window to take the paperwork, and the howling wind rushed into the car. I shuddered. After I filled out the paperwork, I called the number again, and the woman came back out and led me inside to a waiting area. I was suffocating behind my mask, the decrease in oxygen making me feel as if I was exercising.

A few minutes later, I was taken into the upright MRI machine. I had never seen one before. It looked like two gigantic washing machines standing next to each other, with a seat in the narrow space between them. The MRI tech instructed me to sit down and then adjusted the seat to the proper height for the MRI magnets to look at my neck.

I was given earplugs to put in and asked if I would like anything on the TV. I said ESPN would be fine, though I wouldn't be able to see it well. I was instructed to tilt my head back as far as I could in a position that I could hold for twenty minutes or so. Then the tech blasted the volume on the TV and left the room. The MRI started and began clunking loudly as electricity rapidly pulsed through the metal coils, creating the magnetic field needed to obtain the images of my cervical spine.

I felt as if I was in a torture film. Not only did I have trouble breathing with my head in that position, but the MRI was like having a terrible DJ playing his worst EDM hits at 150 decibels in an echo chamber while *SportsCenter* was blaring in the background. The earplugs did little good as the thumping nearly rattled my fillings loose. If I didn't have CCI before, I was sure to have it after this torment.

I got through the extension series and was told I could relax. Thank god. An adjustable bar was then put in front of my face, and I was told to flex my neck as far as I could. My forehead rested on the bar to keep it still as the MRI began its rhythmic door-slamming. My heart rate was sky-high. I could feel my heartbeats between the clunking sounds of the machine.

After what seemed an eternity, the thumping stopped, and the TV noise took over. The tech lowered the volume and came in.

"Sorry, we didn't get what we needed. You have to try to stay still, Dr. Gallagher," she said.

Goddammit, I thought I was staying still. "Okay," I said, "I can give it one more try."

She left and the techno beat began again. I suffered through it, staying as still as I could.

"We got what we needed," she said after coming back in several minutes later. "Thank you. One series left."

"What?" I said, panicking. I thought I was done.

"We still have to get the neutral position images."

"Forget it," I croaked. "I already had those on a static MRI. That's all I need."

"Are you sure?" she asked.

"Absolutely," I said. I was cooked.

She led me out to the waiting area, where I stayed until my images were put on a disc. I retrieved them, drove home, and went to bed, feeling even worse for the next several days. The radiologist contacted me a few days later with his report — no evidence of instability or cord compression. Just some arthritis between the vertebrae. I was disappointed that there would be no surgical fix to my problem, but I was not surprised. At least I had the peace of mind knowing I was not missing something.

Having ruled out CCI, I was left to consider my options. I was on board with what Dr. Bonilla from Stanford recommended. But had I left every stone unturned? Was there anything else I hadn't considered? Possibly, but I needed to follow one path and see where it took me. Certainly, I was not going to follow Mayo Clinic's recommendation of just exercising more.

Months after my visit, Mayo Clinic removed recommendations for graded exercise therapy and cognitive behavioral therapy from their chronic fatigue syndrome webpage. I'm not sure whether this decision stemmed from a change in philosophy and treatment regimen or pressure by the ME community, but it was a small victory for people living with ME nonetheless.

Graded exercise therapy with cognitive behavioral therapy became highly controversial after a study referred to as the PACE trial was published in 2011 in the *Lancet*, one of the world's most renowned medical journals. The authors suggested that ME patients who felt sick after exercise simply needed to advance their activity more carefully. Furthermore, they claimed that cognitive behavioral therapy by a psychotherapist would allow patients to ignore their symptoms so they could be more active. Unfortunately, this study influenced the way many large healthcare and governmental organizations regarded and treated ME, including the CDC, Mayo Clinic, and even my employer. Patients felt they were being gaslighted by those who espoused the PACE trial's recommendations.

The study was later derided publicly for its abundant methodology flaws. Its claim that ME was essentially a psychological illness was discredited in academic circles and scorned by legions of patients on social media. Serious doubts were cast on the results of the study. Ironically, it probably shed more light on ME than any noncontroversial study or public campaign could have at that time.

In 2015, the Committee on the Diagnostic Criteria for Myalgic Encephalomyelitis/Chronic Fatigue Syndrome via the Institute of Medicine published *Beyond Myalgic Encephalomyelitis/Chronic Fatigue Syndrome: Redefining an Illness*. This publication defined new diagnostic criteria for ME. It also proposed a new name, systemic exertion intolerance disease (SEID), though its use has not become widespread. It stated that ME is a serious, debilitating condition that causes significant impairment and disability but that there is no known cause or effective treatment. Readers were cautioned to avoid labeling or misunderstanding ME as a psychological illness, as has been common for decades. This report helped reify ME in the medical community, where skepticism was, ironically, at its apex. Further, the World Health Organization removed chronic fatigue syndrome from the "mental and behavioral disorders" category and created a new diagnostic code for it under "other disorders of the nervous system," called 8E49 post-viral fatigue syndrome.

ME is now most commonly characterized by three major diagnostic criteria: significantly impaired activity level compared to before getting sick, post-exertional malaise, and unrefreshing sleep. These symptoms must be accompanied by either cognitive impairment (aka brain fog) or orthostatic intolerance (worsening symptoms upon standing, as in POTS), or both. Other symptoms not required for diagnosis but commonly reported include pain, sore throat, swollen lymph nodes, sensitivity to lights and sounds, nausea, and headaches.

My symptoms did not meet the diagnostic criteria for a long time. I do not know if that is because I have an unusual case, because I was extremely fit when my illness began, or because the diagnostic criteria don't allow for atypical presentations. I am confident there are plenty of people like me who are early in their illness and therefore do not have all the required symptoms. I believe these criteria accurately capture most ME signs and symptoms, but perhaps they are too stringent. Post-exertional malaise alone, for me, was so severe it was life- and career-altering far before I had unrefreshing sleep or orthostatic intolerance. Did I not have chronic fatigue syndrome until those symptoms manifested? I certainly feel that I did. While these diagnostic criteria may not capture every patient who has ME, in my opinion, they are still the best set of criteria available and a huge improvement from prior standards. I only wish I was diagnosed earlier and that someone had warned me that continuing my intense exercise could be permanently detrimental to my health.

Chapter 19

Largo

We left Rochester and started our journey home with me feeling vexed about my situation. Along the way we visited the murder site of George Floyd. It was just a month after his killing. It put some things in perspective.

We parked two blocks away, just beyond the cement barriers that blocked off the streets. Melissa pushed me in my wheelchair in the late-June heat and humidity, giving me a unique perspective at waist level. We were struck by the powerful nature of the ad hoc monuments that were erected, painted, and chalked around the exact spot where the police officer had kneeled on Floyd's neck. There were thousands upon thousands of once-fresh flowers now dried out in the summer sun. Black and White people alike quietly wandered around the car-free intersection of Thirty-Eighth Street and

South Chicago Avenue. I struggled with the idea that people wanted their picture taken at such a painful memorial site. This was not a tourist trap. It was a murder scene.

As we turned to head back to the car, Owen said to Reese, "Isn't that Mackenzie from school?" Reese turned her head and was momentarily confused. We were a thousand miles from home, and standing there was one of her classmates. We briefly said hello and asked why she was there. Her father, an acquaintance of ours, said hello and explained their summer plans. He tried in vain to hide his confusion about why I was in a wheelchair as his eyes darted from my wife's face quickly down to me and back up to her. I felt an impulse to stand up and show him that I wasn't paralyzed, but I remained seated, saying very little. The all-around heavy experience stuck with me.

We left Minneapolis the next morning for Keystone, South Dakota, just a few hours south of where my bike trip to the Badlands had been. I thought of the road I had been on since then, full of twists and turns, a stark contrast to the long, straight, easy highway we were on. I set the cruise control and relaxed. The bucolic, wide-open plains I-90 runs through allowed me plenty of time to reflect on the disappointing experience I had at Mayo, the grim times of the past six months, and what my future may or may not hold.

An hour into the state of South Dakota, I saw red and blue flashing lights of a Police Interceptor in my mirror. I pulled to the side of the highway, not really caring if I got a ticket. At that point a traffic ticket seemed so meaningless. A female officer got out quickly and approached the passenger side of my car. I rolled down Melissa's window and began to say hello.

"Do you know how fast you were going?" the officer asked.

I knew exactly how fast I was going. I had set the cruise control eight miles per hour over the speed limit in hopes of making good time while avoiding a ticket.

Before I had time to reply, she said, "Can you step out of the vehicle and come back to the patrol car?"

As I followed her back to her police car, she glanced at my wheelchair in the back of my SUV. Because I was looking at her, I stepped into the drop-off between the asphalt and the gravel on the side of the road, twisting my ankle and stumbling but staying on my feet. Once we got into the squad car, she ran my license and told me that because the speed limit was 80 mph, she couldn't be lenient. I sat in the passenger seat of the patrol car, listening to the large German shepherd panting in the back seat as it paced back and forth. Without further discussion, she gave me a written warning and told me to be mindful of the speed limit. I thanked her and walked carefully back to the driver's seat, wondering if her warning was a result of her seeing my wheelchair and my stumble, or perhaps it was a turning point in my seemingly terrible luck.

We pulled into Keystone and checked into our motel room, whose balcony had views of George Washington's face up on Mount Rushmore. We then set out to the National Memorial for the lighting ceremony that evening. We parked in a handicap spot in the parking deck, and Melissa and the kids took turns pushing me up the hill to the entrance, making our way through the crowd of visitors up to a spot where I could see. As the kids wandered about, Melissa stroked my hair and rubbed my shoulders while people glanced at us, studying her good looks and me in my wheelchair. She sat on my lap as the national anthem began to play and the presidents' faces were lit up for the night.

The following day we drove to Crazy Horse Memorial, a mountain carving similar to Mount Rushmore but on a far grander scale. The memorial, which broke ground in 1948, pays homage to the famous Lakota Sioux warrior. It was far from completion but inspiring, as were the stories of its construction. Our day continued with a drive along Needles Highway, a nauseatingly windy but scenic road through the Black Hills surrounding Mount Rushmore, more akin to my personal journey than I-90 had been.

Throughout June, both before and after our trip to the Midwest, I looked for ways to be outside after so much time indoors. I began to use Reese's electric scooter to get out of the house. On good days I had enough energy to ride the scooter a mile up the street and back. It felt euphoric to be in motion. And it got me out of the house and away from thinking about my troubles for a few minutes.

As the summer solstice approached and the weather grew warmer, I also drove to trailhead parking lots and sat in the car with the windows down. This eventually led me to Buckingham Park, a parking lot in Lefthand Canyon next to its eponymous creek, just outside Boulder. The creek is a pastoral fissure running through the rocky landscape that carries snowmelt through the canyon mouth out onto the plains, headed for Nebraska and the South Platte River, on to the Mississippi River and ultimately into the Gulf of Mexico. The creek wound peacefully along the canyon floor until September 2013, when a thousand-year rainfall, as they called it, swelled the rivulet to an inconceivable torrent that dragged massive amounts of mountainside, houses, and roadways with it.

The damage from that flood was still visible at Buckingham Park, but the beauty remained. Because there is only one hundred feet or so between the parking lot and the creek, it was a perfect place for me to get out into nature without expending too much energy—at least after the first few times of going there, when walking down to the water and then back up the gentle grade caused an energy crash. The sound of the rushing water and frothy rapids were spellbinding. My time there offered me a refuge from the constant feeling of being sick, but not from the dark thoughts I had about my illness, which ebbed and flowed as I sat transfixed, staring at the water.

I contemplated ending my life at that exact location. My suffering was not too much to bear in the moment, but I was growing weary. As sick as I felt, I couldn't fathom how others had hung on for years and decades if they felt even worse than this.

I channeled Viktor Frankl some days and searched for meaning in my illness and all the troubles in my life. It was hard to find. Other days I imagined shooting myself in the head, standing at the edge of the creek so that I would fall backward into the water. No one would have to clean anything up. My kids wouldn't be the ones to find me. The paramedics and coroner wouldn't have to deal with a terrible mess. Just a soaking wet, lifeless body with shorts and flip-flops to hoist up the bank of the creek.

My saving grace was that over the summer, my constant nauseated, flulike, hangover state began to recede largo.

I noticed a morning or two per week that I awoke without crippling discomfort or the need to eat quickly. Some days that would last only until after digesting breakfast. Other days it would last until nearly noon. Each time it happened, I considered it a victory and a small step forward. Each time I felt worse, I viewed those days as the calm before the storm. One day I told myself I was sure to get better; the next I was fucked for life. Melissa continued to urge me to "think positive," but I didn't need a life coach. I needed someone to rub my back and cry with me. She was doing the best she could. Nothing and no one could provide me the comfort I sought. Not my wife, not my kids, not my mother, not my twin brother. Only a miracle worker could ease my pain when the darkness hit.

Trouble sleeping seemed to exponentiate the deep, dark dread I was feeling. I finally got to the point where I needed help. For the first time in my life, I asked for an antidepressant. I read conflicting reports about antidepressants, specifically, SSRIs and chronic fatigue syndrome, so I asked my doctor from Stanford about it. He wanted me to stick to the medication he had prescribed to help tease out what was working and what was not, but my depression was too severe. It was unlike anything I had ever experienced. Ultimately, he gave in, and I started taking a low-dose SSRI.

As with all medications, I had immediate side effects. My stomach reeled for the first few weeks, but not quite like the nausea I got from my ME. If the Inuits have fifty words for snow, I was on par with them for ways I could feel sick to my stomach.

The SSRI was also known to cause sexual dysfunction, specifically, delayed ejaculation. For a person with post-exertional malaise, it was an unwelcome change. Sex with my wife had become difficult enough already from the fatigue and malaise. I wondered if others with ME were having the same issues, so I searched online until I found a poll that lent some insight. Of 136 respondents with ME or fibromyalgia, 90 percent reported a decrease in frequency of sex since being diagnosed, three-quarters reported a great impact on their sex life, and more than a third expressed reluctance to have sex because of post-exertional malaise.

So on top of the physical health problems, I now added sexual and psychological health problems to my list of symptoms. There was hardly an aspect of life that chronic fatigue syndrome was not affecting.

Chapter 20

Northport Point

By July, I needed a break from the kids and a change of scenery. Even the creek became too familiar after spending hundreds of hours there. I had enough energy to manage another cruise-controlled road trip by myself—this time to Michigan, where Kevin had a new lake house. If I was tired, I would pull over and sleep in the back of my car or in a hotel. Sure, I was concerned about getting from my car up to a hotel room without exhausting myself, or getting a flat tire with no one to help replace it, but I needed to prove to myself that fear would not dominate my life anymore.

I set out alone in my Kia Telluride, a car I had purchased brand new just weeks before I left work. I drove to Omaha and stayed in the same hotel we had stayed in as a family on our way to Minnesota in June. This made it all the easier, knowing exactly where to park and how far I had to walk. The following day I drove to Chicago, just seven hours, where I would stay the night in another hotel.

The third day I drove the rest of the way to Northport Point, a quaint private golf course community on a peninsula jutting into Lake Michigan at the top of Grand Traverse Bay. Kevin's house was just down the street from the house his wife's grandmother owned since the 1950s. The community had around one hundred cottages, most of which were enough home for two families. Each cottage was adorned with a sign out front with the name of the family that owned it. Most of those families had been coming to Northport and attending sailing and tennis camp there for generations. Everyone seemed to know each other or were quick to introduce themselves and explain their connection to the community.

Not wanting to hold Kevin or his family back, I spent hours each day alone in my bedroom, staring out at the clear, inviting water or resting to restore my energy. The porch off the family room downstairs provided a beautiful perch to take in the lake, as well, though I had to repeatedly explain to passersby that I was not Kevin, the same way I had explained it to Mr. and Mrs. Langenberg a few months prior in St. Louis. A few times I took an opportunity to ease myself off the dock and into the chilly, refreshing water, enjoying it even though my heart rate shot up and left me panting for minutes afterward. I watched with both joy and envy as Kevin pulled the kids behind the Jet Ski on a giant raft around the harbor. Afternoons, we would take a ride around parts of the bay in the boat or through the neighborhood on the golf cart. Being in motion was my salvation.

Despite spending time with family in a serene setting—or perhaps because of it—I struggled each day thinking about my life. Melissa and I texted about the toll my illness was taking on me and the family. The antidepressant was helping me from having the dark thoughts of ending my life, but I was still filled with despair. I couldn't even go to the grocery store. On bad days, I couldn't stand long enough to cook, but if I didn't eat, I got sicker. I read online accounts from other people with ME who would buy chopped vegetables because they couldn't expend the energy to cut them. They would sit on a stool to cook. They would load dishes straight into the dishwasher or leave them out until they had the energy to wash them. I felt pathetic.

After six months of abstaining from alcohol because it made me feel ill, I tried drinking beer to relax and forget about my problems. Alcohol intolerance is practically a required diagnostic criterion for ME according to many who have studied and treated people with the illness. I wondered if alcohol's effect on the GABA receptors of the central nervous system—neurotransmitter receptors that stop or slow neurons—played any role in ME or vice versa. Why was alcohol intolerance so prevalent in ME? Did it drop blood pressure, which people with dysautonomia already have issues with? Or was there some other mechanism? Some days I was able to tolerate a beer, and some days I could not, but I was willing to do anything to get better. Everything got a grade for whether it made me feel better or crash, and beer was no different. So at one point in 2019, I gave it up. The one thing I worried about was that, like exercise, once I gave it up, I might never be able to resume it.

The first evening, I drank half a beer and felt better for about fifteen minutes. An hour later, I felt worse than I had before the beer, but feeling less sick briefly was a relief. I didn't know it at the time, but over the next several months, I would manage to build up a tolerance to a couple of beers—and it actually made me feel better. Perhaps my recovery allowed the alcohol use. Perhaps the alcohol use sped my recovery. It was impossible to know.

Four days into my visit to Michigan, I went for a five-minute walk outside the house. I'd read stories of people who had recovered from the deepest depths of misery with ME— several who couldn't get out of bed for months—who could walk for five or ten minutes at a time. I had told Kevin back in March that if I could just walk for fifteen minutes each day, I would pull through this thing. That lasted no more than a few days and left me housebound. Desperate to resume any sort of walking, I was determined this time to be extremely cautious. I had no choice, anyway.

With walking being this difficult, I wondered how I would ever be able to operate again—which requires standing for hours, often while wearing a heavy lead apron. I had to lift, push, and pull limbs to get bones back into place—bones that many times were reluctant to go back. Even before I became sick, it was routine for me to finish surgery at least somewhat fatigued and hungry, with my scrubs soaking with sweat in the shape of the lead apron.

What a change from where I had been just three years before, I thought. Going for a short walk would now be a victory if I didn't crash in the hours and days afterward. Controlling my urge to ramp up too quickly would be a challenge. It had been my downfall before. I could not trick myself into believing I was capable of more than I was. Pacing was going to be the key to my return to some semblance of health and well-being.

Chapter 21

Leadville

I got home from Michigan at the beginning of August—the month of the Leadville 100 in the Colorado mountains. That August, the race, like most other sporting events, was canceled.

In the years since the onset of my illness, I began to give back to and stay a part of the trail-running community, even when I wasn't able to run. I had taken countless gels and water cups from aid station volunteers over my years of racing, so it was time to repay the favor. In 2017 and 2018, I signed up to help at the Leadville Trail 100 Run, also known as the Race Across the Sky because of its extreme altitude. It is a one-hundred-mile running race and one of five hundred-milers in the Grand Slam of Ultrarunning, making it one of the most revered and popular ultrarunning events. It happens to take place a few hours from Boulder, in the town of Leadville, Colorado.

Leadville is an old mining town that reinvented itself after the Climax Molybdenum Mine closed in the early 1980s. Two locals, Ken Chlouber and Merilee Maupin, created the race to attract tourism to the area. It has since grown into a series of races for both running and mountain biking, and in many ways, put Leadville back on the map.

Both years, I drove up to Leadville the morning of the race and continued on to the even tinier town of Twin Lakes, population 196. I found my place in the firehouse, posing as the Twin Lakes Aid Station, where we would be cooking up hot food before handing it out with gels and drinks to the runners. We also spent time outside the firehouse helping runners find their gear bags, which they had checked at the start of the race. These bags contained the ultramarathoners' preferred nutrition, warmer clothes for changes in the weather, new shoes and socks, and any number of unique personal items—lip balm, toilet paper, bug spray, etc.

Runners headed through the aid station forty miles into their one-hundred-mile mountain trail run. From there, they forged the chilly waters of Clear Creek, hiked or ran up to 12,000 feet to the top of Hope Pass, and ran down the other side to the mile fifty turnaround. Then it was back up and over Hope Pass a second time, back across the creek again, and into Twin Lakes before slogging through the night toward the finish.

The first runner through the aid station in 2018 was Rob Krar. Krar is a professional trail runner and one of the most visible guys in the sport. He has a huge barrel chest and a beard so thick and burly that it has its own Twitter account. He has been very transparent about his battles with severe depression, making him a hero in the eyes of some and more relatable than the typical professional athlete to many.

Krar had an injury to the cartilage on his patella and femur that kept him away from trail running for a full year before the race. His knee surgery put him on crutches for several months. It's the kind of surgery I do routinely. It's the kind of surgery after which most human beings don't run again. Ever.

To rehab his knee, Krar took up cycling, a sport that requires less impact than running. He then rode the Leadville Trail 100 MTB mountain bike race, finishing in a respectable fourteenth place. Buoyed by the fitness he felt during that race, he asked the Leadville race directors if they would make a spot for him in the one-hundred-mile run just *one week* later. He did the seemingly impossible, not only finishing the race after not properly training for it (i.e., not running), but he won, besting the second-place finisher by over an hour. Krar sped so quickly through Twin Lakes to the sounds of cowbells ringing and fans cheering, he was but a blur to everyone there.

I met a more mortal athlete twenty-eight years of age who came in a few hours later, just before dusk. He wore running shorts and a sleeveless shirt. I grabbed his gear bag for him from the numbered pile and helped him unpack as he sat on a plastic folding chair outside the firehouse. The air was starting to cool, and soon enough it would be downright cold. I checked his headlamp for him, filled his bottles with water, and asked what else I could help him with. Then, with little concern in his voice, he asked me, "Is it supposed to rain tonight?"

I couldn't believe what I was hearing. The preparation required for an amateur athlete to run a hundred miles is astonishing. Yet, here was a racer sixty miles in, looking comparatively fresh, without a clue whether he should have packed a rain jacket or warm clothes. On one hand, I envied his youthful athleticism and Pollyanna outlook. On the other hand, I pitied his naïveté and the long night he had ahead of him. He left seemingly unfazed and headed through the tiny town and up the trail's steep switchbacks at the end of the dirt road just a few hundred yards away. He would go on to finish in just over twenty-five hours, a coveted mark that bears the reward of a large finishers' belt buckle that reads UNDER 25 HOURS. In the trail-running community, one-hundred-mile belt buckles supplant the medals hung around marathoners' necks. It's a badge of distinction that can also become part of one's wardrobe.

The next athlete I helped barely beat dusk in the race back to Twin Lakes from Hope Pass, which is no easy task. Unlike the guy I had just sent off, she was prepared for the weather with plenty of layers. What she wasn't prepared for, though, was the dark. She had forgotten to put her headlamp in her gear bag. There was no forging ahead without one.

I hurried around Twin Lakes pleading with other racers' friends and family for a headlamp. Some offered batteries. No one seemed to have an extra headlamp. The runner debated proceeding without one, but I warned her not to do that. As word spread, the trail-running community came to the rescue with a headlamp for her to use. She promised to bring it to the awards ceremony after the race to return it. The crazy thing is that the person who lent it to her probably expected that to happen—and it probably did. Trail runners were just a different breed.

As night fell, the largest wave of runners came to Twin Lakes cold and wet from the creek crossing. Just before the 10:00 p.m. cutoff when racers would not be allowed to proceed further, the aid station was abuzz with runners of all types. There were odd mountain folks with tape-patched jackets and trekking poles who seemed to be speed walking the entire hundred miles; crunchy guys with dreadlocks who could be mistaken for buskers on Pearl Street in Boulder; bulky women with Ironman tattoos on their calves; and a rare few with specially labeled race bibs who were aiming to attain the title of Leadman or Leadwoman—which required completing five Leadville events in one year: a 10K, a fifty-mile bike or run, a marathon, a hundred-mile mountain bike race (the week before like Rob Krar), and the one-hundred-mile run.

Volunteering in Leadville made me feel proud to give back to the running community. It also gave me a larger feeling of loss. Once I was too sick to volunteer, I realized that running a marathon, much less a hundred miles, would be reckless to even consider if a miracle came along and I was able to exercise again. Eventually, I was so ill that I hardly cared about such things. I just wanted to feel healthy.

Before I left Leadville in 2018, I saw a bumper sticker that read FUCK THIS . . . LET'S GO TRAIL RUNNING. I took a picture of it and thought, *How I would love to have the health to go trail running.* I would quit my job and give away all my money to be able to say, "Fuck this," and go for a run. I didn't ever need to race again. I just wanted to feel the freedom of gliding down the trail through a stand of aspen trees turning bright red, yellow, and gold in October, my legs effortlessly making their way past each other with each powerful stride.

Most people race hundred milers to find themselves or test their mettle through unthinkable exhaustion and suffering. It is purely self-imposed. Those people actually pay good money to do this.

Thanks to ME, I didn't have to pay to do this. I saw a side of myself that I didn't know existed. When I was healthy, I felt strong, invincible, and independent. Sometimes I acted that way—even at times in my marriage. When I became sick, I buckled—not the good Leadville 100 kind of buckle, mind you. I lost my edge. It took nearly six years, but once I got so sick that I had to leave work, I folded. I became fearful. I was incapable of going it alone. Not only could I not take care of myself physically, but I also needed someone to help me emotionally. I had muscled my way through medical school, residency, work as a surgeon, deathly hot Ironman races, friends dying, and years of frustration not knowing what was wrong with me, but I found my breaking point. Being that sick was soul crushing. Not knowing what my future would look like in a month bankrupted me mentally.

SEPTEMBER IN THE GALLAGHER HOUSEHOLD MEANS KIDS back in school and NFL. Two thousand twenty would be no exception, even though things would look a little different. The kids would be home again due to COVID, and I would gradually return to walking short distances at the beginning of football season.

What we look forward to even more than school and football, though, is jarring tomatoes. Each September, before the leaves begin to fall from our fire-engine-red sugar maple in the backyard, we set up camp in the garage and driveway and prepare to jar the following year's supply of tomatoes and sauce, the way that Nonina taught Melissa to do. Melissa buys roughly two hundred pounds of tomatoes from an organic farm. Delicious, organic San Marzano or Roma tomatoes are not as easy to find in Colorado as they are in other parts of the country. Each year is a new hunt to find out which farm has tomatoes available to the public, what condition the tomatoes are in, and when they will be ripe.

We keep our calendar open in September to jar the tomatoes when the tomatoes tell us they are ready.

Our kids love the tradition. They invite their friends over to witness and take part in the festivities. Those friends' parents usually come by, too. We often celebrate finishing the job with dinner and wine outside. That time of year is perfect in Colorado. There is always a small chance for freezing weather, even snow, but most years it is gorgeous. The kids have turned down going on vacation just to jar tomatoes.

My duties typically include getting down all the heavy equipment from the shelves high up in the garage, washing the buckets, paring the tomatoes, running the cooked tomatoes through the press, and boiling the jars. Melissa helps pare the tomatoes, then cooks them for the press and makes sauce that we jar in addition to the tomato puree. With my fatigue, I let the kids and Melissa do the lion's share of the work and supervised the kids, who did more of the physical labor than they had in years past. But at least I documented more with my camera than I had been able to before. We got all the work done, even if it wasn't as smooth as usual, and it reminded me of a silver lining I hadn't considered before.

I developed ME at an age that allowed it to steal a lot from me. Had I developed it at twenty, though, it would have stolen even more. I may never have had the career I had or made a family. If I had gotten ill in my fifties or sixties instead, I may have lost less in terms of my career—but perhaps without the strength to fight it. I am thankful that my kids were old enough to have seen their dad be active before becoming so sedentary. They were also at an age where they could express compassion for my plight, which was heartwarming and helped me get through a few very dark days. The worst of my illness coinciding with COVID-19 was also a mixed blessing. Because our kids were home from school, we grew closer as a family in many ways. We also drove each other nuts. Seeing a parent fight through an illness and all its challenges can be a valuable lesson even if the illness doesn't go away.

With the slow improvement in my condition, I had planned to go back to work on November 2. Before returning to work, I went back to see Dr. Silver, who continued to follow my progress and manage my illness through my visits with Mayo Clinic and Stanford. I felt reassured when she agreed with Stanford's diagnosis and plan, helped me fill their recommended prescriptions locally, and added a few things to the plan herself. It was like a spoonful of medicine knowing how much she cared and how smart she was. Even though I had looked for more answers and verification elsewhere, I trusted everything she did for me. We had a partnership in decision-making about my health. She understood what it takes to be a surgeon just as much as she understood what it takes to race an Ironman.

As November approached, my paid sick time had run out, and my disability insurance claim was taking far longer to process than I had anticipated. I needed income, and I wanted to get out of the house. The problem was, our work schedule was made three to four months in advance to allow for clinic and operating room assignments. In my situation, it meant trying to predict my health that far in advance. It was impossible.

Ultimately, my fatigue kept me from returning for even the three half days a week I was scheduled to work for the rest of the year. My partners felt the brunt of my absence. Schedules had to be juggled. People had to cover my shifts. The

January schedule, which was made before I realized I wasn't coming back in November, had me in the operating room two half days that month. That meant that for my return on January 4, I would have an OR scheduled just three days after my ten-month absence.

No rest for the weary.

Chapter 22

Falling Off a Log

While I was sick, I had plenty of time to think about my illness. Too much time. I obsessed about it. My thoughts were as unhealthy as my body. I began to think about trading illnesses. Would I rather have ME or multiple sclerosis? I would list the pros and cons. My neighbor had had MS for fifteen years, and I saw her out jogging on occasion. Some patients with MS have remissions, and life is more or less normal. I knew that wish was unrealistic, though; I'd had tons of wheelchair-bound MS patients with brittle bones that have broken just transferring to bed.

I'd also amputated a lot of legs over the years—most from people in ill health, but a few who were otherwise healthy and vibrant aside from a mangled foot or leg caused by an accident. I said out loud, "I'd rather have a below-knee amputation than have this." After all, I had seen Dave Mackey, whose leg was amputated after a boulder crushed it while trail running, finish the Leadman competition, including a finale of completing the LT100 in under twenty-five hours, netting him not only the larger buckle for the hundred mile run but a personalized trophy—a pickaxe with the word LEADMAN burned into the handle.

I considered other illnesses and disabilities: paraplegia, cancer, complex fractures. I told Melissa at one point, "If there was a pill that gave me a 50 percent chance of being completely cured and a 50 percent chance of dying, I would take it right now." What I didn't know at that time was whether the suffering was going to get worse or ease up. It was incredibly discomfiting to be fearful of dying yet have thoughts of risking my life or suicide.

These thoughts were counterproductive. There is no sense in comparing suffering. Someone with paraplegia might be downright offended or deeply wounded to hear that a person with ME would consider their situation any better. Many would consider it insensitive. The fact is, I wasn't thinking clearly. I was desperate and despondent. I have witnessed the same type of response in my patients to their own maladies.

Before leaving work, I had patient after patient show up in my office with tears in their eyes. A few cried throughout most of the visit. Because of my own suffering, I was baffled by how someone who had torn their ACL could be crying about it. Didn't they know that with our modern surgical techniques, it was more than likely that they could still bike and swim and even run? I was unable to do any of those things. I would trade places with them in a New York minute.

But that was not possible. Nor was it how I truly felt. I knew they were suffering just the same as I was suffering. It meant a change in their lifestyle. Or it meant their plans were ruined. Some had plane tickets to travel. Others had bowling leagues that were their entire social life. Many were depended on to work to support their family. A few were primary caretakers for sick, elderly spouses or parents.

I kept that in mind when I explained the treatment plan for any injury, and my patient review scores were never higher. Despite the fleeting thoughts about my own illness, I found it far easier to keep the spotlight on the patients as I was taught to do. It was helping me as much as it was helping them. When you're suffering inside, looking outward to help others can be effective medicine.

My time off also helped me become more relatable. Once I took my leave of absence, I let my hair grow out. I wasn't seeing patients or colleagues, plus my hairdresser was not working during the COVID shutdowns. I had considered growing it longer before, but I was too self-conscious; I never wanted a patient to feel uncomfortable with my appearance. I wanted patients to take me just as seriously as I took my job.

Being serious about patients' problems is important, but so is being relatable. Once I honed my surgical and clinical skills, becoming more confident in the process, I was able to let my guard down a little, making a joke here or there if I was sure it would land right. Mostly, though, I remained determined and focused, aiming to be compassionate at the same time. I kept my hair short and dressed conservatively. Eventually, I started growing a beard in the winters and was delighted that my patient reviews went up. No patients ever seemed to mind, and a few told me they liked it. By late winter, it was pretty thick, but not like that of ultrarunner Rob Krar or the baristas in Boulder's cafés. Come summer each year, though, the beard had to go.

As my hair grew longer during my time off, my kids began to complain about it. "Seriously, Dad, are you going to keep your hair long?" they'd say. "You look like a weirdo." I was amused that my kids were more conservative than I was. Or perhaps they didn't want their dad posing as a fellow teenager. They begged me to get it cut. Eventually, I caved in before returning to work, getting it neatened up but not short like it used to be.

DURING MY FIRST WEEK BACK TO WORK, PEOPLE TOLD ME how much they missed me and how glad they were to have me back. It was heartwarming. I felt appreciated. I was happy to see so many people I missed and to be out of the house after so long, though it was an adjustment not spending my days with Melissa anymore.

A couple of the other surgeons came to my office, welcoming me back and offering to help in any way they could. It was great seeing Jeff, who was closing in on his last day in practice. Lance was there to check in on me constantly and offered to protect me if anyone gave me a hard time about my limited schedule. "Tell them to fucking talk to me if they do," he said. Another one of my partners, who had been covering for me when any of my patients had questions by phone or email, made sure I didn't need any help in the operating room.

Thankfully, all my initial surgeries, which were not very complex, went well. It felt easier than coming back from some of my vacations. When I operated with Jeff fixing a hip fracture, he was astonished that I hadn't missed a beat. "Like falling off a log," he said. It was the last time we ever operated together. He retired a week later.

Even with all the positivity surrounding my return, I grew anxious answering questions about my illness. I was not ready to tell people I was struggling with chronic fatigue syndrome. Those words were so hard to get out. "I have dysautonomia," I said, or, "It's a neurological disorder." Because I wasn't upfront about my condition, though, rumors abounded. Some heard I had cancer. Others heard I had a neurological disease, which was somewhat true. I suppose it is natural for people to make assumptions when someone suddenly disappears from work for nearly a year. I felt like I had to address the situation.

So I spoke with Kevin and Kelly to get their opinions. I told them I was considering writing a letter to my partners about my diagnosis to avoid answering any more questions, but also to shed light on the condition. Kelly suggested to me that because I was a doctor, I had the perfect platform to promote research and understanding of ME. With their full support, I wrote an email and sent the draft to them for approval. They looked it over and thought it was great. Then, I hit send. In doing so, I shared my diagnosis and a succinct explanation of what ME truly is with my colleagues in the department of orthopedics, not knowing how they'd respond. I immediately felt relief that it was out there, but I worried what effect it would have on how people saw me.

The response was by and large fabulously supportive. It was reassuring to get such positive feedback from my partners. A few people I didn't expect to reach out to me shared their appreciation and confessed their misunderstanding of the illness. Some stopped me in the halls at work and told me they were impressed by my courage. I was truly humbled.

As a result, I sent the email to several hundred primary care physicians in hopes that they would learn from my experience about the stigma and lack of understanding surrounding ME. I posted a copy of the email along with an introduction on Medium.com and got back on Facebook after a four-year hiatus to share a link to the Medium article and a fundraising link for #MEAction. The response I got on Facebook was overwhelming. High school friends, medical school classmates, and other people I had lost touch with reached out to me. A few weeks later, #MEAction sent out a series of tweets quoting my article and linking to it. I hoped that those who read it gained a better understanding of ME —or an understanding at all—to help get the ball rolling on destigmatizing it.

Overall, it was great to be back at work, and I felt relieved now that people knew about my condition. But it wasn't all roses. One of my partners accused me of cherry-picking easy cases. Another surgeon from another campus said, "Your partners were not very happy about having to pick up the extra work while you were gone, but welcome back." She had a track record of spewing claptrap, so I tried to let her words fall like water off a duck's back. It was sometimes hard to do that, though.

Being vulnerable and sharing with others was terrifying. When we expose our weaknesses and insecurities, we fear that people will judge us harshly or ignore what we are saying. People usually respond poorly either because they are uncomfortable with what they are hearing or because they do not know how to respond and therefore appear apathetic —

perhaps because they're wrapped up in their own struggles, have selfish interests, or are just oblivious to the needs of others.

Being back at work meant having to be alert and ready to make important decisions. To help clear my head each morning, I began getting up very early again to stretch and meditate. I couldn't exercise, but I did what I could to show up as sharp as possible. Unlike years past, when I would wake up before my alarm went off to exercise, review my work schedule, and email colleagues, I did not simply spring out of bed anymore with a fear of missing out.

In many ways, my career and my athletic endeavors were built from a fear of missing out on doing something remarkable with my life. I was scared of mediocrity. I also had a formidable fear of failure. I still do. I was not born to be a surgeon. I saw going to medical school as a way to achieve something great.

Getting through medical school was not on my radar when I left high school. Becoming a surgeon and doing a fellowship at Harvard was beyond my wildest dreams. So was qualifying for Boston and racing Ironmans. I didn't dare to think that big when I was younger. As life progressed, I realized I wanted to do great things, not average things. My childhood idol, Bernie Lynch, was perfectly content to stay in his blue-collar job and simple house. I wanted to be content with a simple life, too, but I chose a different path, shooting for the stars instead. I never considered why. Bernie's greatness was his ability to enjoy life and be content, not constantly seek more. I still want that, but I haven't achieved it. ME has renewed my focus on that slower-paced, simpler lifestyle in some ways. Being able to stand at the sink and do the dishes without feeling sick is fucking awesome. But so is staying at the Four Seasons or traveling to Europe. I'm a work in progress.

Chapter 23

Long Haulers

During my absence from work, news coverage ramped up about COVID long haulers. Long haulers are people who have gotten over COVID but continue to have post-viral symptoms, much the same way that those with ME develop long-term symptoms following other viral illnesses. These lasting symptoms, like chronic coughing and shortness of breath, were recognized early in the pandemic. The Infectious Diseases Society of America refers to the condition as post-acute COVID-19 syndrome.

The *Journal of the American Medical Association* (*JAMA*) published a survey of 177 COVID patients who self-reported symptoms several months after their acute infections. Around one in eight people reported fatigue as a persistent symptom.

This was found in patients who had both mild and severe COVID symptoms initially. Brain fog was reported by a small number of people, as well. Further studies have documented these symptoms, along with pain, heart palpitations, dizziness, and more, making the constellation of symptoms eerily similar to those that people with ME have been dealing with for decades.

Given the massive number of people in the United States and worldwide who have been infected with COVID, this could translate into millions of people globally with long COVID symptoms.

The hope in the ME community is that long COVID will shed much-needed light on the disease. As dreadful as COVID has been for so many people who have lost their lives, their loved ones, their livelihoods, and their businesses, it is possible that the pandemic advances the medical understanding and awareness of ME.

The popular press has glommed on to COVID long haulers. A *60 Minutes* special that aired in November 2020, "Puzzling, Often Debilitating After-Effects Plaguing COVID-19 'Long-Haulers,'" featured several athletes, including runners, before they were infected with COVID. After their infections, which did not necessarily require hospitalization, they developed headaches, blurry vision, fatigue, brain fog, malaise, and more. They went from being active, fit adults to having trouble with activities of daily living. The special also featured New York physicians who established a clinic to evaluate, research, and treat these patients. One of the physicians taking care of patients in this clinic had long hauler symptoms herself.

Long haulers are being taken seriously, thank goodness, although that is not universally true. One primary care physician who had read the email I'd sent at work about my diagnosis confessed she had dismissed a patient with this constellation of symptoms after COVID, not knowing what to make of the woman's complaints. There is still a lot of progress to make.

The *New York Times* has repeatedly covered COVID long haulers. One article that featured individual long haulers was entitled, "What If You Never Get Better from COVID-19?" The tagline is "Some patients could be living with the aftereffects for years to come. Recent research into another persistent, mysterious disease might help us understand how to treat them." A picture of a woman with her twelve-year-old daughter laying her head in her lap is shown with a caption that reports that the two "still have symptoms, including severely elevated heart rates, shortness of breath, and debilitating fatigue." The mother called it "a nightmare."

These symptoms sound hauntingly familiar to the utterances of the #MillionsMissing: *I got a virus and never got better*. Dr.

Fauci has commented on the similarities between long-hauler symptoms and ME, which has sparked optimism that more money will be spent trying to understand the cause and treatment of both, if they are in fact different and do not share the same mechanisms of disease.

"We Are Everywhere." It's a phrase I used to see on bumper stickers of Volkswagen Buses and other vehicles driven by Grateful Dead fans who subscribed to their brand of counterculture. It was a reference to Deadheads being ubiquitous from rural America to the big cities and from any station in life. When I saw that furtive reference, I felt like part of something bigger than myself, part of a community that shared a common experience. It was the same way I felt with my CrossFit community.

People living with ME are everywhere, too. After sending friends the email about my battle with ME, I received several responses from people who either had been diagnosed with ME or had an uncannily similar story, but felt lost in the shuffle of the healthcare system and didn't yet have a diagnosis. It opened my eyes not only to just how many lives this touches but also to how alone many who live with ME feel. My email served to make some of them feel they were finally part of a community with similar experiences to theirs, much the same way I felt when embracing the ME community online and on social media. It's much more personal when there is only one or two degrees of separation from you and someone else dealing with your illness. I have felt a sense of relief each time I have heard from someone whose brother or sister also suffers from ME because it adds legitimacy to my own story.

One such person, whom I went to elementary school with and hadn't heard from in more than two decades, reached out to me, admitting he'd been sick for ten years and was still suffering. "I'm really glad we connected," he wrote, "because it gives me some real hope. That's something I haven't had in a while."

A medical school classmate shared that she had been suffering from depression and had to take a leave of absence from work because of ME. She had been too ashamed to admit it publicly and called me brave for sharing my story publicly. I told her that during the toughest part of my battle with ME, I developed terrible depression. I had not made that part of the story public until now, because like ME, mental health issues have a stigma attached to them.

Like depression, ME is also considered by far too many people as a condition of weakness. Patients are treated as though they are lazy, malingering, or imagining their symptoms, so they don't receive a proper diagnosis—a fast track to depression and second-guessing oneself. The resulting depression may become apparent, leading friends and family to attribute the illness to being all in their loved one's head. It is a vicious circle.

Adding to this kind of thinking is that ME is invisible to lab tests. There is no MRI or blood marker at this point that can rule in or rule out ME. The clinician must take the patient's word for it. Some of us have POTS or dysautonomia that leads to measurable irregularities in blood pressure or heart rate. I felt reassured in many ways that I had a documentable tachycardia with changes in posture or minimal exertion, but many do not. Without a test to prove the diagnosis one way or the other, many physicians will dismiss the patient as difficult or dramatic or nuts.

For an unknown reason, women are victims of this more often than men, which also causes the "hysterical" label to be used. Multiple sclerosis was once considered a psychological disease, referred to as "hysterical paralysis," in large part because middle-aged women were the typical patient. Men, who dominated the field of medicine for much of the twentieth century, were quick to blame the patient or assign a diagnosis, rather than looking deeper into the situation. It is a matter of human nature and arrogance for many doctors to feel that if they cannot figure out the diagnosis, then surely the patient must be feigning their symptoms or exaggerating otherwise mild complaints.

I have fallen prey to this in my own clinical practice. Part of that was likely my own hubris, part of that was feeling guilty that I couldn't solve the patient's problem, and part of that is the system at large. Doctors are given precious little time with patients today. As an orthopedic surgeon, though, I have the benefit of seeing a lot of problems that are obvious; the X-ray, MRI, or CT scan tells it all. That is one of the beautiful parts of orthopedic fracture management. A broken bone is often a very straightforward diagnosis. Understanding the problem is the easy part in those situations. Knowing what to do next—cast or brace or surgery—is more sophisticated. Having the skills to fix the problem surgically is why we train so long. But elucidating the situation to the patient is often the hardest part and the one that we get very little training in.

I spend far more time explaining to patients why they do not need surgery than why they do need it. Our society has become obsessed with quick fixes to just about everything, and surgery is not immune to this. We have become so good at solving problems surgically that we are victims of our own success. With increasing frequency, we have patients now walk—or crutch or wheel—into our offices, expecting a pill or surgery to fix everything and restore things to the way they were the very moment before they were injured.

When the diagnosis is not clear, we as physicians struggle. If we cannot see it on an MRI, then surely there is nothing wrong with the patient's shoulder, right? Perhaps we can find someone else to shuffle the patient to. Shoulder pain can emanate from the neck, so we'll look there and hope there is something visible radiographically that allows us to send the patient to the spine surgeon. If not, we'll send the patient to the physical therapist and let them deal with it for a few months. If that fails, we can try a steroid shot in the shoulder and see what happens. When all that fails, blame the patient. The next patient is waiting and probably has a real problem we can see on an X-ray.

This type of thinking is all too common, even if it is subconscious. Many of us cannot bear the guilt of failing to help the patient in their time of need. So, we use these picayune tactics to absolve ourselves from the responsibility of having to look deeper into the problem or admitting that we simply do not know the answer. I work in a closed system, meaning we do not send patients to physicians outside our group except under certain less common circumstances. That means the buck stops with us. We must figure out the problem ourselves. There is no "expert" we can dump the patient on when the diagnosis is unclear, or the treatment is too difficult. *We* are the experts. That leaves my colleagues and me in a position where we must answer the patient's questions to their satisfaction and treat their problems without looking for someplace else to refer them to. It is a system that I believe has helped me and many of my colleagues be better clinicians.

The same is true for post-acute COVID-19 syndrome. My primary care colleagues will be the final stop for many long haulers looking for answers. My hope is that each of them recognizes what these patients are telling them and can use the valuable lessons we have learned from ME to help treat them. Perhaps, like ME patients have figured out, the answer is to stop, rest, and pace.

Chapter 24

Who Will Dance with Me?

On Valentine's Day 2021, a month and a half after my return to work, I decorated our bedroom with neon pink and green hearts that I cut out of construction paper and hung from the eves of the vaulted ceiling that extended in a Y-shape on either side of the chandelier. Melissa was over the moon about it. When she opened the door and saw the hearts, she started screaming with joy. Nine hours later she was screaming again, but this time with grief.

While we were standing in the kitchen at her friend's house that night, Melissa saw a missed call on her phone from her friend Mikey—part of a group of guys she called her "Philly boys."

"That's weird. Mikey never calls me," she said. She then got a text from Mikey, telling her to call him. He had bad news. Their close friend Chris was dead.

"What! What are you saying? What? What?" she screamed over the phone. "What do you mean? I just talked to him Friday. What?" I had never seen her so distraught.

Chris was a close friend of Melissa's and the centerpoint in her Dave Matthews Band circle of friends. Melissa met Chris years before at a Dave Matthews concert. He was a towering figure, standing six feet three inches and weighing 260 pounds—about the size of my father when I was a kid. Unlike my dad, Chris wore a smile everywhere he went, accompanying it with a number 3 Allen Iverson Philadelphia 76ers jersey and a yellow Seattle Sombrero hat at all three-hundred-plus Dave Matthews shows he'd been to. Fans everywhere knew him. Dave Matthews himself recognized Chris repeatedly at his concerts and would hold up three fingers as a shout-out to Chris and his number 3 jersey.

Melissa and her girlfriends traveled with Chris and his guy friends from Philadelphia over the years seeing Dave Matthews concerts around the country together. I first met Chris at a DMB concert, just after I got sick in 2014. A year or two later, Chris, his wife, and their kids stayed at our house for a week in the summer. We got to know each other better, sharing stories and seeing a moose together for the first time up in the Indian Peaks Wilderness just above Boulder.

Chris and his wife were wonderful parents. Chris was also a middle school guidance counselor, and he offered Melissa advice a few times about helping our kids when they were bullied. Chris had a magical ability to capture the attention of those he spoke with and made the people he engaged with feel like they were the sole focus of his attention.

Melissa had grown closer to Chris after a medical emergency he had a year and a half before his sudden death. Chris seemed to return to good health by New Year's Eve 2020, and he sent out a video saying goodbye to all the problems of 2020 and wishing a prosperous 2021 to all his friends. "Who will dance with me?" he asked, then played Dave Matthews' "Grace Is Gone" and began to show his moves. His children got up and danced with him. His wife walked in during the video and joined in, too. Just six weeks later, he died suddenly.

Melissa took the shocking news as hard as I have ever seen her react. She discussed the devastating loss with her girlfriends, Mikey, and the rest of the Philly boys over the coming days. They played Monday morning quarterback, wondering what went wrong and whether there was anything they could have done to prevent his untimely death, though there was not.

Melissa and I talked for days about the senselessness of it all. Several times a day, she would burst out crying. I felt like crying myself. The year that had given me the worst my life had to offer was now preying on my loved ones.

self centered

Chris's death was not the only tragic news we would get that week.

Six days after Chris's death, I got an email from my dear friend Luke's mother, Mary. It said that Luke was in the hospital. He had fallen the night before while his kids were at his house, and he lacerated his scalp. He started bleeding profusely and was unresponsive. His children called 911. Luke was taken to a hospital just a few miles away and intubated. Worse, he was in liver and kidney failure. Mary told me Luke had been drinking heavily for a while and had tried to hide it, but she and her husband were aware that he was in bad shape. They had tried to get him help, but he refused. They had plans to go up to see him once they were vaccinated in another two weeks.

"I am terrified," Mary wrote.

I quickly called Luke's father, Henry, to speak with him and Mary about Luke's condition. Over the past couple of weeks, Luke's skin and eyes began to turn yellow with jaundice. He wore glasses and grew a beard to conceal it. Kevin and I had been talking and texting each other with concerns about Luke's drinking over the past several months. We had also spoken about it with our close friend Frank, our old roommate in Boulder, who was living near Luke and saw him frequently.

None of us thought for a second that he was in bad enough shape to have liver failure at age forty-seven.

Luke's marriage ended in spectacularly bad fashion several years before. "I just can't trust her," he told me.

He said he offered to work things out with his wife, but she didn't seem interested. Luke told Kevin and me that because his wife had been handling all the finances, he was surprised to find out that they were in significant credit card debt when they separated. Luke spent a vast amount on attorney fees for the divorce proceedings, which he felt was worth it in the end. He stayed in their house after the divorce, and they split custody of the kids. But he never got over the failure of the marriage.

His wife had driven a wedge between Luke and his parents before the divorce. Henry and Mary lived just a block away and were as helpful with the grandkids as any grandparents could be. Luke's wife convinced him that his parents were overbearing, though. She was awful to them, they said. Eventually, Henry and Mary moved down south to be close to their other son, Carter. Luke and his kids did not speak to Henry and Mary for several years until Luke realized how furtive his wife had been and sought their counsel. Being the great parents they had always been, they were there for Luke when he needed them.

At one point after the divorce, Luke seemed happy. We kept in touch on a WhatsApp group we titled the Cranford Fan Club, named after our ToastChee-eating friend from high school in North Carolina. The group included Luke, Kevin, Vincent, Cranford, and me. We sent pictures and text messages nearly daily, humoring each other, discussing Vincent's plethora of girlfriends, or just catching up. A year or two after his divorce, Luke began dating, then living with a new girlfriend and sent us pictures of them together for more than a year. Ultimately, that relationship faltered, too. Worse, Luke lost the job he'd had for more than fifteen years, followed by the next two he tried his hand at. He seemed to be okay early in 2020. Despite the pandemic, he was reporting to the Cranford Fan Club that several women had spent the night with him from time to time. That summer he visited his brother, who noticed how gaunt he looked. His muscles were wasting away. Luke admitted to me on the phone in 2020 that his legs felt so weak that he couldn't run and even went to the doctor about it the year before. I began to wonder if he had some neurological issue he wasn't telling us about or whether his drinking was getting out of hand. He denied having a problem, telling us that he never drank at home anymore.

We last saw each other in November 2019, before my health hit rock bottom. The Cranford Fan Club had scheduled a trip to stay at Vincent's house on Scotland Cay in the Abacos, the easternmost chain of islands of the Bahamas. Vincent's father built the house two decades prior, just before dying of brain cancer. Vincent's stepmother kept the architectural gem on the private island, letting her boyfriend use it as a fishing shack for years until she passed away and Vincent inherited the worn-down edifice.

On a reconnaissance trip to the house he met John, a man about his age who was renting a neighbor's house. Vincent struck up a deal with him. John could fly his plane from Florida over to the island and use Vincent's house whenever he would like, so long as he fixed up the place. John turned it into something special over the ensuing years. The Cranford Fan Club was excited to finally see it for the first time.

Cranford and Luke both hesitated to go, wary about the tiny airplane required to get us to the island. Eventually, peer pressure won, and we all bought tickets. Two weeks later, Dorian, a Category 5 hurricane, flooded the island, removed every leaf from every shred of vegetation, and destroyed Vincent's house. The roof was ripped off. The walls were gone. Waterlogged mattresses and couches were piled up in the kitchen. The appliances were barely recognizable. The before and after pictures showed little resemblance to each other.

The Cranford Fan Club would not be thwarted by one Cat 5 hurricane, though. So, with two weeks until the trip, Kevin and I asked Kelly if we could rent her house in the swanky Ocean Reef Club on Key Largo. Kelly and her husband, Tiff, being incredibly gracious as always, said yes. Kevin and I agreed to do it with some reservations, knowing that the Cranford Fan Club members, despite closing in on fifty years old, can be very rowdy and even destructive at times. We feared Tiff might never speak to us again if we wrecked his vacation home.

We convened in Miami, and Kevin, Luke, and I stayed one night at the opulent 1 Hotel. Kevin's company had business relationships with the owner, so he could get us a discount on the astronomical prices. We had been there a couple of years before with Luke, who charged everything he could to the room the three of us were splitting. That included a $40 tube of sunscreen, which sold for around $5 across the street at the drugstore.

He spent money like a Rockefeller, despite having gone through an expensive divorce and a pay cut. He polished off a liter of Jack Daniels easily and had to buy a pint to keep the party going before the long weekend was over. That was the first time I considered he might have a drinking problem, but his behavior was never out of control. He provided ample entertainment for the weekend. He got us out on the water, rented Jet Skis, talked random women into having their pictures taken with an orange Ping-Pong ball he carried around with him, and told nonstop jokes.

This year was no different. Luke ordered two double vodka martinis in the first hour we were there, along with plenty of food from the poolside bar. Kevin, being sober and paying for a third of the hotel bill, was less than amused. But we were lifelong friends, and the kid had been through a lot of tough times lately, so we both tried to shrug it off.

After our brief but expensive stay in Miami, we made our way down to the Ocean Reef Club. Cranford flew in and followed us there in his rental car down the long, unswerving two-lane road ensconced with mangroves on both sides. Getting through the front gate of the community was harder than getting through US customs, thanks to the club's stringent rules. Kevin and I were admonished during a visit years prior for running shirtless, even though we were doing so before sunrise. The chances that one of the Cranford Fan Club members would break the etiquette rules were as likely as one of us breaking a window or a lamp in my sister's house.

Once at the house, we divvied up rooms, unpacked, and then took the golf cart over to the village market, where we stocked up on food and drinks. Vincent was still out on the Abacos, surveying the damage to his house. He would join us the next day.

Our first evening at Ocean Reef, we laid low and made dinner at the house. The air was warm, and we spent most of the evening out back, in and out of the pool, catching each other up on our kids and jobs. After chatting for a while, I noticed that Cranford had been standing waist-deep in the pool for several hours.

"Are you going to stay in there forever, Cranford?" I asked.

"Ah, dude. This pool is awesome," he assured us. "Why would I ever get out?"

Cranford put his beer down on the edge of the pool, leaned back, and floated into the deep end, his round white belly half above the surface of the water aimed skyward. I laughed and thought how nice it was to enjoy a quiet night without kids in warm, humid air with a pool and good friends. Cranford floated around happily and then made it back to his beer. The skinniest kid in high school, he was now closer to 230 pounds and could tolerate a few drinks. He finished his beer and asked Luke to go in the house and get him another. While he waited, he started making guttural sounds and babbling to himself. I began to wonder if he really needed another beer and whether we should put a life vest on him.

After Luke came out and handed Cranford a beer, he turned to Kevin and me. "That's his fifteenth beer."

"No way!" I said. "He only bought a twelve-pack."

"Go look," Luke said. "The bottles are in the recycling."

I went inside and was astonished that Luke was right. Where the hell did he put fifteen beers? I would be dead if I drank fifteen beers, even Michelob Ultra, which was all Cranford would drink. We decided it was time to coax Cranford out of the pool and call it a night. Vincent would be there the next day anyway, so we had to save our energy.

I assumed Cranford would be in bed the whole next day nursing a hangover, but to my surprise, he was his usual self by 8:00 a.m. I sneaked away to my bedroom and meditated, then came out and did my handstand and air squat routine.

"So, what's going on with your health, dude?" Cranford asked, watching me. From time to time, I would mention to the guys on WhatsApp that I was feeling sick and didn't know why.

"I still don't know," I answered. "I have to conserve my energy these days. If I do too much, it wipes me out and makes me sick."

"Man. That sounds serious," he said.

"I'm looking for answers, but I haven't found anyone who can really help me."

"That's just fucked up," Luke offered.

"At least I can still work," I said, not knowing what the coming months would have in store.

Vincent got there later that day with plenty of beer and vodka along with a friend of his from Argentina. Mariano, a heavily cologned psychiatrist who vaped constantly, was charming, sincere, and a genuinely nice guy. We probably scared him with our rowdy, crass behavior. Then again, he was friends with Vincent, so he probably knew what he was in for.

The boys of the CFC managed not to destroy the house, but Kevin and I spent half our time there cleaning up, doing dishes, and vacuuming. Kevin was a good sport about recycling all the beer bottles everyone else left around.

The second day, we hired a boat to take us out snorkeling. At 8:00 a.m. we met our captain, an attractive twentysomething who wore short shorts with a bikini top. We headed out to the century-old lighthouse sitting on the coral reef a few miles offshore. After our captain anchored near the metal structure, we jumped into the water and found ourselves surrounded by all kinds of marine life—everything from eels to barracuda. Luke got out of the water early while the rest of us used up every minute we could exploring life underwater. When we got back to the boat, it was apparent that Luke was more interested in the captain than any of the pelagic wildlife found with a snorkel and mask. His libido was still as intact as the imperishable lighthouse.

That evening after a few beers, things started to get a little unruly. Crude jokes started flying back and forth. We started roasting one another, bringing up each other's foibles and recalling past embarrassing incidents. Then it happened.

Vincent pulled out one of his testicles and walked around the pool with it exposed, coming out of the Velcro fly opening in the front of his bathing suit. We all laughed. "Look at the size of this!" he exclaimed. "That's just *one* of them. There are *two* of these!"

While he paraded around the pool, Vincent got perilously close to Luke. "Get the fuck away from me, man," Luke warned him. Vincent smirked and took a step closer, then *whack*. Luke hit him in his exposed testicle with the back of his hand. Vincent fell to the ground.

"*Ohhhh. Ohhhhhh*," he groaned, holding his hands over his groin as he lay curled in a ball.

"I told you not to get near me, man," Luke said.

Vincent roared, "That *reeeeallly* hurt. *Ohhhhhh*. . . . Do it again!"

We died laughing. Vincent was insane. He always had been.

"You're fucked up," Luke said, staring down at Vincent, who was still writhing around on the ground with one ball out of his swimsuit. Luke wasn't angry, but his stern look was enough warning for Vincent to cut it out.

Vincent and Luke made amends with each other by smoking pot shortly afterward. Luke, obviously stoned, pulled out the Bluetooth speaker he brought with him and started playing music. I started to mess with him by changing the music with my phone's Bluetooth setting. Luke got confused and tried to put his music on again. I changed it again, and he got more confused. After he reset the music once more, I changed it a third time.

"What the fuck is wrong with this thing?" he said, getting pissed.

I started cracking up. Luke realized it was me messing with him and hurled the speaker at me. Hard. Really hard. It struck me square in the chest. A foot higher and it would've seriously injured me or knocked me unconscious. Kevin leaped out of his chair and screamed at Luke, aiming to protect me and Kelly's house.

Realizing what he had done, Luke burst into tears. He wrapped his arms around me and repeatedly apologized for an awkwardly long time. The mood of the evening had suddenly and dramatically changed. Luke wiped away the snot and tears with a pool towel and went to bed. The rest of us sat in silence for a few minutes.

"Well, that was fucked up," Vincent said. Poor Mariano didn't know what to say as a new friend or a psychiatrist.

The next morning Luke didn't show his face till nearly noon. We all reassured him that everything was cool, but he kept apologizing.

"Here, Michael, it's yours," he said, handing me the speaker.

"I certainly don't want it," I said, shaking my head and holding up my palms in a *not me* gesture.

"Well, I'm leaving it here, then," he exclaimed. "Someone else can take it."

"Give it to Vincent," I recommended.

"Sure. I'll take it," Vincent said, smiling as he accepted the speaker.

Since that trip, we have bantered constantly about being angry enough to throw a speaker at someone. Luke accepted that his anger was to blame for his actions. But he didn't address the underlying issue. It would ultimately get the best of him.

Chapter 25

Happiness Is Being One of the Gang

Over the course of the next year after our rendezvous in Key Largo, Luke began to drink more than usual. Like most alcoholics, he hid it well for a while. Later in the year, Frank told Kevin that Luke looked unhealthy. After Kevin and I started noticing that he was sending fewer texts and pictures—and that the few he did send revealed sad eyes behind the blue light filtering glasses he had started wearing all the time—we worried that something was going on. Perhaps the isolation of COVID and his lack of employment were taking a toll on him.

Even with our concerns, when his mother emailed me, I was stunned to read that he was in the ICU. Even if he was drinking excessively, I did not expect him to end up in the hospital in sudden liver and kidney failure. This was his first hospitalization. The alcoholics I have known personally and taken care of professionally often have multiple trips to the hospital for drinking-related mishaps before getting to this point.

I spoke with Luke's parents, his brother, Carter, and Frank, trying to find out all I could. The doctors said his bilirubin—a breakdown product of old red blood cells that a healthy liver clears from the bloodstream—was as high as they had ever seen, indicating that his liver was badly damaged. His kidneys totally shut down, as well. He was put on constant dialysis through a vein in his neck to make up for his renal failure. He was sedated and on a ventilator. His dangerously low blood pressure required pressors to keep the blood flowing through his organs. Apparently he had vomited and aspirated the contents of his stomach into his lungs, further complicating the situation by causing pneumonia and sepsis. He was too unstable to transfer to a university hospital for a higher level of care.

Over the ensuing days, Luke remained sedated and on the ventilator. His kidneys failed to recover, and he made precious little urine. His liver function suggested he had acute alcoholic hepatitis and possibly irreversible cirrhosis. He required three medications to keep his blood pressure up. The critical care doctor told me that to evaluate his mental status, they had to stop giving him sedation and pain medications.

It took nearly a full day for him to respond at all. Eventually, he started biting at the endotracheal tube that provided him respirations—a sign he was not brain dead. The following day, his mother told me that when she spoke loudly next to Luke's ear, he turned his head once. Another day he squeezed her hand. But he wasn't opening his eyes. To look for evidence of seizures from alcohol withdrawal, which can be present even without obvious physical signs, the doctors performed an EEG. Thankfully, there was none.

Because of COVID, Mrs. Phillips was the only one allowed in the ICU. Luke's brother, whom Luke had designated his medical power of attorney, and his father could not go in. So Mary took pictures for them and FaceTimed them so they could see him and so Luke could hear their voices.

I feared Luke would die. I wondered if he would need both liver and kidney transplants, but I wasn't sure if he was even eligible, given his medical status and the amount of alcohol he had been drinking. Current alcohol use disqualifies most alcoholic patients from getting a liver transplant. They typically need to prove abstinence for a period of time before being approved for a new organ. Still, I had to do something. So after Luke was admitted, Melissa and I began to make phone calls to find someone who could help. The kid who held onto my belt loop to keep me from falling out of a moving car while I was high on kind bud in high school was now hanging on by a thread himself.

Unfortunately, my suspicions were right. One of the liver transplant programs we contacted had a hepatologist, who was willing to accept him to their ICU once he was stable and could prove he could maintain sobriety, but the program's ICU doctor refused. We had no way to force their hand. Luke was too sick to survive without a transplant yet not a candidate to have a transplant unless he could survive awhile without one. At his relatively young age, it seemed so unfair.

We tried three closer large hospitals that performed transplant surgeries across the river in another state. An ambulance could get him to one of the hospitals in under thirty minutes. But because Luke had not worked in a while and had Medicaid in another state, the nearby hospitals were not likely to get paid for any surgery they did on Luke and were unwilling to take him.

After six days languishing at the hospital, Luke was showing no signs of improvement. His mental status seemed to worsen, perhaps from the high levels of ammonia in his blood or the bleeding in his brain.

"We have to call the university," I said to Melissa.

Instantly, she picked up the phone and began putting her superpowers to work.

"Can I have the transplant team, please?" she said to the hospital operator. She was routed to a voicemail. She called back again. Same result. She called a third time and got through to someone on the transplant team.

"This is Melissa Gallagher. I am trying to get a patient to your hospital for a transplant." She got right to the point. "He is at a community hospital, and he is going to die if he doesn't come there."

The person she was speaking to was in charge of coordinating accepting livers from deceased patients. He was clearly not the person who could accept someone needing a liver. He would have someone else call her, though. Fifteen minutes later, Melissa spoke with the liver transplant coordinator and got the phone number of the attending transplant surgeon on call. The coordinator would make the attending aware of the situation. We then spoke with Luke's ICU doctor and gave her the phone number. We knew there were no guarantees. Luke's mental status was an obstacle. His insurance was an obstacle. His hemodynamic instability was an obstacle. His alcoholism was an obstacle. Still, we had to do everything we could to try to save his life.

Luke's ex-wife brought his children over to his house to see their grandparents and uncle, who explained the situation and told them he may never come home again. It was an agonizing task. At fourteen and seventeen years old, the kids were able to understand how serious Luke's condition was and recognized that alcohol was the culprit. To make matters worse, his kids were not allowed to see him at the hospital.

Mrs. Phillips then made a trip across town to explain the same to her 102-year-old mother. Four generations of Phillipses were pulling for Luke. So was the Cranford Fan Club. "Come on, Luke!" we each wrote. I posted a picture of a Peanuts pillowcase Kevin and I had as kids that said HAPPINESS IS BEING ONE OF THE GANG.

I spoke with Carter the next day after he had visited Luke's house. Letters and bills filled his mailbox. It was so full that the post office had stopped delivering to it. Carter said Luke hadn't checked his mail in nearly two months and had scores of voicemails on his phone dating back to 2017, many from people asking him how he was doing.

How much pain had he been in? Why did he not ask for help after pleading with me to do so when I was sick and depressed? As I gave updates to the CFC, the other guys sent their exasperated responses. Vincent seemed especially upset. His close friend had died on his front porch in a chair facing out at the rain in Pucon, Chile, just four months before from the exact same battle with drugs and alcohol. Like Luke, his organs shut down. I couldn't fathom how many people I knew whose lives had been affected directly by substance abuse.

Dr. Patel, Luke's overseeing physician in the ICU, updated Carter and me on several occasions, most often detailing Luke's lack of improvement. She had a soft, youthful voice with an Indian accent. I guessed that this was her first job out of a critical care fellowship by the way she comported herself on the phone. She had started a seven-day stretch of covering the ICU the morning after Luke's admission. I detected a hint of the strain in her voice, likely imparted by having a young, critically ill patient who was not responding to medical treatments. She was at the helm of Luke's care. We had to rely on both her clinical skills as well as her willingness and ability to convince another hospital to take him. She had been told no so far. I wondered if she was being aggressive enough to get him transferred.

I also wondered if she was going through the same things I went through early in my career—namely learning to be assertive for the sake of the patient, despite opposition. More than that, I prayed she was being as hypervigilant about details as possible to save my friend's life. One of the details she needed to be paying attention to was ammonia.

When laypeople think of ammonia, they think household cleaners. When hepatologists think of ammonia, they think liver dysfunction. The liver is responsible for clearing toxins from the blood. Toxins, like ammonia. Ammonia is produced in the body as a waste product of protein breakdown, usually from digestion. The liver turns ammonia into urea, which is excreted in the urine.

Ammonia can also be produced from skeletal muscle breakdown during intense exercise. When I lived in North Carolina, I remember the distinct smell of ammonia emanating from my pores after runs in the hot sun. For the sick, increased levels of ammonia in the blood can cause problems in the brain. These problems include swelling (cerebral edema) and increased pressure (intracranial hypertension). Both can lead to brain damage and even herniation of the brain, leading to death. This is one way patients with liver disease can die. *Hepatic encephalopathy* is the global term for brain dysfunction related to liver disease and is common in patients with acute liver failure. This can manifest in personality changes, cognitive dysfunction, and even loss of consciousness.

When people have high levels of ammonia, a medication called lactulose is used to try to rid the blood of the ammonia by decreasing how much the intestine produces and absorbs ammonia. It also causes people to have bowel movements to excrete the ammonia. Too much lactulose, and people are stricken with life-threatening diarrhea, so the medication must be titrated until the ammonia level comes down. If too much lactulose is given, the diarrhea can cause dehydration or electrolyte imbalances.

For Luke, his ammonia levels remained high for days after his admission to the hospital despite being given lactulose. It clouded the picture of his mental status. When his sedation was turned off and he remained unresponsive, we questioned whether he had permanent brain damage from the ammonia and the bleeding around his brain. If that were the case, would it be worth living?

After a week, however, Luke's ammonia levels started to drop. He began to follow simple commands and eventually opened his eyes.

Adding to the stress of Luke's situation was that Liam found out Luke was sick. He was angry that no one had told him for six days that Luke had been in the hospital. Kevin and I had debated whether telling him was the right move, but we ultimately decided to focus on Luke and not get distracted by Liam. Liam found out about Luke from someone else, though. He began questioning whether it was true via a series of texts and voicemails. He suggested that Luke was poisoned because he was a super soldier. Liam's fixed delusions were straight out of a Jason Bourne movie. I had heard them for years.

After I realized he wasn't letting up, I gave in and answered one of his calls. I spoke with him for forty-five minutes.

"There is no way Luke drank himself to death," Liam said. "I have been trying to drink myself to death for *years*. And *nothing*. I drink a fifth of vodka seven days a week and an extra handle or two on top of that. Luke is indestructible. You think his liver isn't stronger than mine? He was poisoned. He was poisoned! No doubt about it. Give me his parents' phone number."

"I can't, Liam. They are grieving. They don't need any more stress right now."

"Okay, then give me Carter's phone number."

"No way."

"Are you fucking kidding me? Is he actually in the hospital?"

"Yes. I told you. He's in the ICU on life support. He has liver and kidney failure."

"Bullshit! He fell and hit his head, and that gave him liver failure?"

"No. He was sick and jaundiced. He was weak and intoxicated and couldn't stand up. He hit his head when he fell. They took him to the hospital, and he was in liver and kidney failure."

"Bullshit."

"I love you, Liam, but I have to go."

I hung up the phone. Ugh. How exhausting. Liam called me nonstop for the next eighteen hours, all the way through the night. I silenced my phone.

I awoke to dozens of text messages. They made little sense:

I CAN ONLY PRAY TO HIT MY HEAD, HEART, AND SOUL . . .

ONLY TO BE DISCOVERED THAT MY LIVER AND KIDNEYS ARE
SHOT.

WHO THE FUCK ARE YOU KIDDING? LUKE'S LIVER IS THE
LEAST OF HIS CONCERNS. NOW, IF THEY SAID DICK CANCER
. . . MAYBE I WOULD BUY THAT.

REMEMBER THE BOYZ THAT RAISED YOU.

Then:

1-800-FLOWERS CAN'T EVEN HANDLE THE ORDER I'VE SENT
TO LUKE.

TRUST ME. I WILL FIND THE FLORIST THAT CAN COMBINE
$1,000
ARRANGEMENT.

PROBABLY DIDN'T THINK OF THAT DR. SURGEON.

Then:

HEY CHRONIC FAGGOT SYNDROME! WAKE THE FUCK UP . .
. IT'S TIME TO WORK ON THE LUKE CASE.

Then:

LUKE PHILLIPS WAS POISONED. IF THE ORGAN FAILURE IS TRUE. . . I BET MY RIGHT HAND. METHANOL/GLYCOL. CHECK IT OUT AND LET US ALL KNOW.

LIAM WAS MAKING A HORRIBLE SITUATION EVEN HARDER. He got others involved who knew Luke as kids. I heard from our old friend Red and Liam's sister, Helene. They asked if it was true. I confirmed that it was.

Each of us had read drunken, psychotic, sometimes threatening text rants from Liam for years. Sometimes we were in the same group text. Many of the phone numbers on the group texts were not in my contacts, so I couldn't even tell who Liam was harassing. No one ever responded. None of us believed Luke would be in liver failure before Liam. But here we were.

I heard from Mrs. Phillips every day. On Luke's seventh day in the hospital, she said she was reluctant to leave his side during visiting hours. She told me Mr. Phillips had broken down emotionally, repeatedly, when they were alone. I felt terrible for them. No one deserved this.

Liam managed to call the hospital and convince the nurse to get Mrs. Phillips on the phone. Wisely, she told him to talk to me from there on out. I am sure Liam was sweet to her, but he also likely spewed some conspiracy theory that added to her pain.

Luke's condition was not improving, but he remained relatively stable for the next week. They slowly tried to wean him from the pressors, but had difficulty doing so. He began to breathe on his own while still on the ventilator and was eventually extubated. Just two days later, though, he was struggling to breathe again and had to get reintubated. During his period off the ventilator, he opened his eyes a few times but only briefly. He said nothing. He shook his head when his mother asked him if he was in pain, but that was his only communication with her.

I spoke with his doctors and Carter on a three-way call each afternoon, discussing his condition and his limited options. Melissa spoke with Mrs. Phillips, offering her comfort and support. I could hear the toll it was taking on them in their voices. Mrs. Phillips sent me texts every day, including a couple of pictures of Luke. His skin was simultaneously yellow and ashen. His cheeks were sunken. He was grayer than I'd ever seen him. His dark eyelids remained closed. I sent the pictures and updates to the rest of the Cranford Fan Club.

By day thirteen, Mrs. Phillips started to text me with increasing worry. "For some reason I feel less hope today than any other. His abdomen and extremities look like a blow-up doll," she wrote.

By day fifteen, Luke began to bleed. His platelets had been low, but his liver was still making clotting factors. Blood then began to come out of his endotracheal tube, his nose, and his rectal tube. I suspected he had a condition called DIC, often caused by sepsis, which leads to massive bleeding.

Carter texted me the following morning, telling me that Luke's condition had worsened. The doctor said he was acidotic—that he had a buildup of excessive acid in the blood—and on pure oxygen on the ventilator. His hours on this earth were numbered.

I sent a message to the Cranford Fan Club:

LUKE ISN'T GOING TO MAKE IT MUCH LONGER, GUYS.

Kevin called me immediately, while I was on my way to work. I told him what was happening, choking on my tears as we spoke. When I got to the physicians' parking lot, I sat in my car and started bawling.

"Why do I have so much pain in my life?" I asked out loud.

I held my head in my hands. I wept for the tragedy. I wept for the two children who were about to lose their father and the two parents who were losing their son. I wept for Carter, who was in disbelief that he was losing a brother too soon. After a few minutes, I walked into work in a daze, hiding my teary eyes as I went straight to my office, where I cried more.

After hardly weeping for thirty years, I began crying routinely a year ago—first because of everything ME had stolen from me, then with the onset of my depression, the decline in my mother's health, my sister's troubles with addiction, the scourge of COVID-19, and now the impending tragic loss of my oldest friend.

Luke died at noon, with his parents and Carter at his bedside. He was taken off the ventilator and lasted only a few minutes. Carter called and told me the news. "We both lost a brother today," he said. I broke down in the middle of the clinic, laying my head on the desk and closing my eyes as I let the tears flow.

When I regained my composure, I called Kevin and texted the Cranford Fan Club. In our friend's honor, we renamed it the Phillips Fan Club. Over the next several days, we shared tons of photos and memories of Luke with each other. Seeing the pictures of Luke with Kevin and me when he was two and three years old added to the nearly unbearable pain.

MR. AND MRS. PHILLIPS HAVE BEEN LIKE FAMILY TO ME. I revere them as parents and wonderful human beings. Although the loss of their son is in no way their fault, they still blame themselves and question what they could have done to prevent it. All of us who are close to him have asked ourselves that question. I feel like I missed how much pain he was in. Growing up, Kevin and I were always there to look out for Luke, even though we were friends and equals. Perhaps now as an adult I was too focused on my own suffering as a result of this horrible illness I now know is myalgic encephalomyelitis.

My ME didn't cause Luke to be an alcoholic. Neither did COVID. But both were pieces of the puzzle in his life and mine. The difference is that Luke's puzzle has no more pieces left. I know mine does, and I intend to place each one with extraordinary intention.

Epilogue

The loss of Luke is still difficult for me today. I think about his kids all the time. I talk with his parents and brother periodically. It has brought us closer together as we plan for what we hope will be a celebration of life that is not limited by the never-ending pandemic.

I also think about the well-being of everyone I love who struggles with addiction. My sister Kristi has given her siblings and herself hope that she can and will stay sober. She has started an ambitious career path by enrolling in an architecture degree program. She has a great eye for design and used that in the past for remodeling houses, as well as decorating and staging businesses. Kristi and I recently had our first really meaningful conversation in years, reconnecting a relationship that has been in need of repair.

She is a big part of her daughters' lives again and makes routine trips to see our mom, making sure she has both company and help. The visits are good for both of them.

I am done ruminating constantly about my own illness, though I still do not know if I am going to get better or worse with time, whether my fate will be like those of the #MillionsMissing who are suffering immensely.

I haven't had to use a wheelchair since last summer, and I am extremely thankful for that. I am grateful to be back to work, seeing patients and operating part time. I still have energy crashes every week or two, but they are far less severe than they were in 2020. I am on guard about my illness at all times because if I am not, I will easily do something that makes me sick. I still think about how much energy it will take each time I go up the stairs. I take the elevator at work. I avoid big surgeries that are going to make me ill whenever I can, but my work ethic, ego, and desire to keep my skills sharp sometimes prevent me from protecting myself. I think less about retirement and more about being healthy and happy today or this year. I have a much healthier relationship with money, worrying less about saving and more about having fun and living a remarkable life. This is one of the best things that has come out of this illness for me. I find I have a greater appreciation for everything I have in life.

In many ways, my marriage is better than it ever has been. Melissa and I connect on a level we never did before. My illness has contributed to that. We spend more time together. We lie in bed and talk, sit on the back porch and sip our coffee together, and discuss both the present and the future, focusing so much less on the past.

I still struggle with not being the able-bodied person I once was. I miss running every single day. I dream about it nearly every night. I now have an electric bike with a throttle that allows me to ride without pedaling up into the mountains along the routes I used to power myself up. I feel truly happy in those moments in the foothills among the evergreens, the sun on my face and the wind blowing my hair back.

Like all people with ME, I have to respect and stay within my energy envelope. That envelope used to seem nearly limitless as I raced marathons and triathlons. Now it is finite, with a blurred and ever-moving edge. One day it may mean doing no more than two surgeries. Other days it means not leaving the house.

The light being shined on COVID-19 long haulers has the potential to be groundbreaking for people with ME. Long COVID symptoms are all too similar to be a separate issue that has no overlap with ME. Long COVID may someday be classified as a subtype of ME, but that conclusion cannot be made quite yet. In early 2021, Congress appropriated $1.15 billion to the NIH for research on long COVID, giving reason for optimism among people affected by ME that a treatment or cure may be found. However, the popular press and the healthcare community can already use the clear association between the conditions to help stop marginalizing people who suffer from ME.

The goals I had for myself just a few years ago have vanished. They were crushed by my illness. Perhaps the most uplifting way to describe it, though, is to say my goals have changed. I have been able to adapt to my new set of circumstances and set new goals. It took a while to understand my limitations and come to grips with them, but eventually I discovered what I am now capable of and adjusted my life accordingly. What would life be without attainable goals? No, these are not the goals I wanted to have at this age.

They are the goals I am *forced* to have. There is a sadness that comes along with that, but there is also some freedom. I was chained to some of the goals I had set for myself, often leading to me neglecting other parts of my life. In this moment, I feel fortunate to be able to set any goals for myself. For a decade or more, I dreamed of running Comrades Marathon for my fiftieth birthday with my brother. It is the grandaddy of road ultramarathons, held each spring in South Africa. It goes either fifty-five miles uphill from Durban to Pietermaritzburg or downhill in the opposite direction, depending on the year. That can't happen now. Kevin may run it, and if I am healthy enough to travel, I may go with him. I will not ever think about racing it again, though. If I do get back to the point that I can run someday, everyone who knows me should talk me out of even contemplating running another race, let alone a fifty-five-mile ultramarathon. Perhaps I should have done Comrades when I had the chance, but I could say that about one hundred things.

When I was healthy, I felt like I was packing life full of a lot. I just didn't get to everything on my bucket list. Work and life got in the way. I dreamed of biking around Europe. I have always wanted to learn to surf. I wanted to get strong enough to do a muscle-up in CrossFit. I secured lodging at the bottom of the Grand Canyon to run rim-to-rim with Rod for his fiftieth birthday—twice canceled and now unlikely to ever happen.

My goals now are more pedestrian. In medicine, we have a lot of sayings regarding bad circumstances, because we see them a lot and can only work with what we are given, despite the advances in technology. "You can't make a silk purse out of a sow's ear," we sometimes say or "You can't make chicken salad out of chicken shit." Attempts during surgery to make things better at the risk of making things worse are warned against in training when we are told, "The enemy of good is better."

We strive for perfection and excellence and have to chasten ourselves against unnecessary risks to get there, lest we undo the work that has been done or keep a patient under anesthesia for an unnecessarily long time, increasing the risks of complications. Young surgeons second-guess themselves, spending too long making decisions or trying to fix something that may have no effect on a patient's outcome. As we learn from our mistakes in our careers, not only do we get faster and better at making decisions (including ignoring what distracts us from the best outcome), but we also clearly define our goals before we make the incision, knowing what is possible and what is not based on experience. People with ME also learn from experience what is possible and what is not.

After suffering from ME for more than seven years now, I have had to constantly change my goals. What I was capable of even a few years ago is impossible now. But some things that were impossible twelve months ago are now possible again. I have much to be thankful for.

But I am still a dreamer.

If I had one goal that I could snap my fingers and attain on a given day, running rim-to-rim-to-rim (R2R2R) of the Grand Canyon would be it. I've dreamed of it for years. R2R2R is not a race; in fact, there never will be an official race there, as it is a national park and it is prohibited. That's partly what makes it so alluring. Running R2R2R is done for the sense of accomplishment. It's done for the pure joy of running. It's done for seeing something on a massively grand scale in nature. I had an article about running it on my bulletin board in my office at work for years, but I took it down after getting sick and realizing it was beyond my grasp. I still think about it from time to time, though, and I keep the article in a drawer, too heartbroken and perhaps too optimistic to throw it away.

A more realistic goal for me is to not feel sick all the time. To have enough energy to enjoy my life. My audacious goals would be to go for a trail run once a month or run a few miles a couple of times a week. If I could trade all my life savings to be able to bike up into the mountains at will, I would. Seriously.

Feeling happy and healthy is priority number one at this point, not exercising. I love running like nothing else, but I'd be perfectly content to never run again and just feel normal— perhaps be able to ride my bike down to Pearl Street for dinner, chase my kids around, and not think about whether everything I do will make me sick.

With Reese, I would skateboard, jump on the trampoline, and do backflips and gainers off the diving board again. With Owen, I would ride his Onewheel, bike to school, play golf, and keep running the BOLDERBoulder 10K each Memorial Day. With Melissa, I would go for hikes, have sex without worrying about being too tired or getting sick, and snowboard on deep powder days followed by a few beers on the mountain.

If I were in perfect health, I would attempt to remodel a house myself. In my spare time, I would stop contemplating and start converting a Sprinter van to a camper or restore an old VW 21-window bus. Maybe I'd live the van life one day, traveling from the mountains, where I would mountain bike and trail run to the beach, where I would finally learn to surf. And I would take the victory lap I dreamed of in Boston, undoubtedly smiling through tears at the finish line.

My accomplishments as a result of my illness include finally writing a book, increasing my knowledge of Spanish, learning and practicing meditation, spending more time with the kids, connecting with Melissa on a deeper level, mastering the art of sourdough bread, and reading tons more. I have also gained a more profound appreciation for work — being able to operate and helping others feeds my soul. I spend more time with my patients and see them through the lens of both a surgeon and a patient who has been through trying times.

I have become more open and able to express vulnerability — this book is a prime example. I hated to show weakness in any form before all this. My kids had seen me weep once or twice in their whole lives until the floodgates opened in 2020 when I got so sick. I believe they have learned some positive things from seeing me battle through this. They look out for me, telling me not to overdo it at home when I try to fix a broken toilet or rake the leaves. Yet they still witness me getting up and going to work, providing for the family, and helping other people who need to be fixed.

As a result of my illness, I am much more aware of my own mortality. Many others are more so, too, because of COVID, whether it has taken the life of someone they love or not. Luke's death amplified this for me. It is the deep connections that we make with other people in this lifetime that matter the most and give life its true meaning.

It has been excruciating at times being even more aware of how much each day counts while being unable to live the life I want because of ME. The lesson I am learning is how to be happy in spite of my illness, my limitations, and the trauma I have experienced over the past two years. For people with ME, it can take all the remaining precious energy we have to live a truly happy life under our new circumstances, but I now know we are capable of it with the help of those who love and care for us.

Acknowledgments

The suffering of many contributed to the completion of this book. That fact is not lost on me. That includes my family, my friends, my patients, and millions of strangers who share the same awful illness that I do. You all deserve acknowledgment for what you have been through and may continue to go through. There are far too many people with ME whose suffering is so immense that they have no chance to find a silver lining as I have. The success of this book would mean a better understanding of a much-maligned illness and group of people, the destigmatization of the words *chronic fatigue,* and the acceptance of the name *myalgic encephalomyelitis*, or *ME.*

Christina Roth, it was serendipity finding you. Your insights and ability to see what I was trying to accomplish here truly made this book possible. You are an artist shaping the clay that others stack in vaguely familiar blocks into statues worth admiring.

Kara Goucher, your selflessness giving your time and words to help lend credence and visibility to this book are invaluable. Your name alone will help others take notice and give this book a chance they might not have, otherwise. Your giving spirit is as powerful as your running career.

To my sister Kelly, without your encouragement for me to stand up, say aloud my diagnosis at work, and share my story, this book never would have happened. Your positive spirit through loss and health battles of your own has inspired me and continues to do so. You have become the matriarch of the family, holding us together like glue when each of us has needed every kind of support imaginable. You personify generosity and grace. Thank you, thank you, thank you.

Kevin and Kristi, I thank you for allowing me to share your stories and how they affected me personally. Kevin, we have had laughs and runs and tears and hotel rooms together our entire lives. I am so glad we didn't lose you along the way. I am sorry for everything, and I forgive you for anything. Kristi, thank you for all the years you were patient with me living with you and your growing family on Franklin Street. I particularly appreciate your graciousness in trusting me with your story. I look forward to your book someday and the chapters you will write over the next few years.

Mom, if you've made it this far, that means these stories haven't killed you. You have lived life the right way and taught us all how to be better, kinder, more patient people. I will forever cherish your endless support and the thousands of times you laughed at my life stories and jokes, making me feel like what I had to say was capable of entertaining others. I love you, Mama.

Pops, thank you for providing for us, including our education both in and out of school. I hope whatever it was that was troubling you all those years is over.

Thanks to all the following:

To Jeff Wood for allowing me to share your story, helping pioneer a treatment for those with CCI and ME, and for your personal support of this book.

To Scott Simpson for helping a stranger on a triathlon forum, giving me insight into the power of rest and recovery, and how to navigate life without my beloved running.

To the members of the Cranford Fan Club, I'm sorry if this book makes you famous. It was bound to happen one way or another, anyway. Chat with you on WhatsApp later today.

To Roger for pushing me to race faster, for endlessly talking triathlon and crypto with me, and for being the first to set eyes on what I have written, reading through an unpolished collection of anecdotes yet still telling me I had a story worth sharing.

To Alison for being a friend in the truest sense of the word and making me feel worthy of praise. You know where I come from, and you seem to get where I am going.

To Rod and Adair for helping me get through some of the truly darkest times in my life and for being a source of light, joy, and entertainment in the rest of it.

To Parag for sitting next to me in the lecture halls, shooting the shit, believing in me as a surgeon, and offering curbside consults over the phone for twenty years.

To the real Luke, Carter, Mary, and Henry Phillips, we have laughed and played and cried together my entire life. We will be family forever. Peace and love.

To the real Liam, you will always be my brother, no matter how ravaged you are by the demons you cannot control.

In remembrance of Bernie and Alice Lynch. You are my heroes.

About the Author

Michael Gallagher is an orthopedic surgeon residing in Boulder, Colorado. He has been living with myalgic encephalomyelitis since 2014. He is a former runner and triathlete trying to get back to doing the things he loves most. He and his wife, Melissa, have two children, Owen and Reese.

LEARN MORE AT:

MDGALLAGHER.COM   AMAZON AUTHOR PAGE

 @GALLAGHER80304

/MICHAELGALLAGHERAUTHOR

Made in the USA
Thornton, CO
09/01/22 20:54:34

a1b2d6b2-d066-41f4-bcbe-4c685cf58098R01